MANAGEMENT OF GASTRIC CANCER

Edited by **Nabil Ismaili**

Management of Gastric Cancer
Edited by Nabil Ismaili

Published by InTech
Janeza Trdine 9, 51000 Rijeka, Croatia

Publishing Process Manager Davor Vidic

Technical Editor Teodora Smiljanic

Cover Designer InTech Design Team

Additional hard copies can be obtained from orders@intechopen.com

Management of Gastric Cancer, Edited by Nabil Ismaili
p. cm.
ISBN 978-953-307-344-6

For EU product safety concerns:
IN TECH d.o.o., Prolaz Marije Krucifikse Kozulić 3, 51000 Rijeka, Croatia,
info@intechopen.com or visit our website at intechopen.com.

Meet the editor

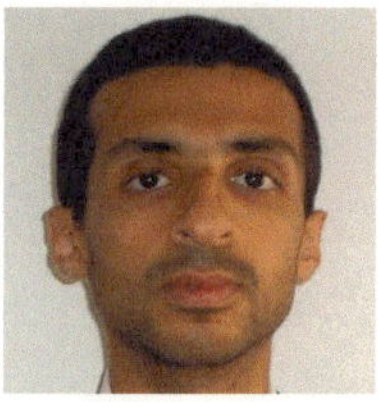

After five years of medical school at Mohammed V University, Faculty of Medicine and Pharmacy and two years of medical practice at the University Hospital in Rabat - Morocco, Dr. Nabil Ismaili joined the department of medical oncology at the National Institute of Oncology in Rabat where he spent four years and the department of medical oncology at Léon-Bérard Cancer Center in France for a one year spell.
The main research areas in which he participated concerned different types and aspects of cancer diseases: breast cancers, urological cancers, and nasopharyngeal cancers. Dr. Ismaili published several scientific papers dealing with concurrent chemoradiotherapy in cancer of the breast, bladder cancer and nasopharyngeal cancer. He is an executive member in various associations in Cancer Research (MEACR: Middle East Association of Cancer Research; ASCAS: Association Scientifique des Cancérologues du Sud). In addition, he has several certificates in different fields of oncology (short trainings in Morocco and abroad). Dr. Ismaili is presently with the Regional Cancer Center of Agadir in Morocco where he serves as a medical oncologist.

Contents

Preface

Gastric cancer is the fifth most common cancer and the second most common cause of cancer death worldwide. The highest incidence was seen in Korea and Japan because of early diagnosis by screening policy. Environmental risk factors include Helicobacter pylori infection, high salt intake, smoking and genetic factors.

Two major classifications are currently used and the Japanese classification is the most commonly used. More than 50% of the patients have advanced disease at diagnosis and in this case the disease has a poor outcome. The diagnosis is confirmed by endoscopy and the histological examination of the biopsy specimen. Adenocarcinoma is the most common histological type. The staging of gastric cancers is based on endoscopic ultrasound, computed tomography, magnetic resonance imaging, positron emission tomography, in addition to the laparoscopic staging.

In localized disease, the surgery remains the mainstay treatment of this malignancy. Many improvements in the surgical techniques have been seen in the last decade. Laparoscopic surgery is an emerging approach which offers important advantages: less blood loss, reduced postoperative pain, accelerated recovery, early return to normal bowel function and reduced hospital stay. However, laparoscopic surgery as a treatment approach to gastric cancer requires further investigations as the extent of lymph node dissection remains controversial. D1 lymphadenectomy, with a goal of examining 15 or greater lymph nodes is a standard. D2 dissection is considered as a standard in several institutions especially in eastern Asia. Perioperative chemotherapy is considered as a therapeutic standard for stage 2 disease. Concurrent radiochemotherapy is also recognized as a standard after surgery for patients at high risk of relapse.

Palliative chemotherapy is the mainstay treatment of advanced stages of the disease (metastatic and non-operable tumors). Several randomized studies have the aim to improve the efficacy and the safety of chemotherapy treatments. The best knowledge in molecular biology has led to the development of new targeted therapies that have improved the results in efficacy and safety.

Despite these treatment advances, the prognosis of gastric cancer remains poor with a 5-year survival ranging from 10 to 15% in all stages combined.

This book provides a real insight into the staging and treatment of patients with this illness that is very relevant to clinicians worldwide. In addition, a chapter has been reserved to a rare type of gastric carcinoma.

Nabil Ismaili, MD
Department of Medical Oncology
Regional Cancer Center
Agadir,
Morocco

Part 1

Gastric Cancer Staging

1

The Role of Computed Tomography in the Imaging of Gastric Carcinoma

Marco Moschetta, Amato Antonio Stabile Ianora, Federico Cazzato, Arnaldo Scardapane and Giuseppe Angelelli
Department of Radiology/University of Bari Medical School
Bari
Italy

1. Introduction

Gastric carcinoma represents the most common gastric neoplasm accounting for 95% of all gastric tumors (Angelelli et al, 2001; Fishman et al, 1996; JH Kim et al, 2006; Levine & Megibow, 1994). Besides, it is one of the most common cancer in the world and a major cause of morbidity and mortality. It cause 30% of the cancer deaths in high risk areas, such as China and Japan. The peak of incidence of gastric carcinoma is estimated from between 50 and 70 years and its prevalence is variable in different countries. This pathological condition has a greater impact in certain geographical areas, such as Japan, Latin America and Eastern Europe. In fact, the prevalence of gastric carcinoma is very high in Japan, where the mortality rate is about 110 cases/100.000 inhabitants while a value of 50/100.000 has been estimated in Italy. Males are affected more commonly than females, with most patients presenting in the sixth decade.

Gastric carcinoma represents an aggressive tumor with a 5 year survival rate less than 20% (Lee DH, 2000). Superficial carcinoma forms are called "early gastric cancer" and have a better prognosis, with a 5 year survival rate of more than 90%. In fact, the 5 year survival rates range from 3% in case of stage IV to 85-90% in case of stage I, depending on tumor stage (Ba-Ssalamah et al, 2003; JH Kim et al, 2006).

Among etiological factors, some dietary habits have been identified, such as hot or salty food. Unlike the esophageal carcinoma, alcohol and smoking do not seem to influence the incidence of gastric carcinoma. Atrophic gastritis, gastric ulcers, intestinal metaplasia, reflux esophagitis, gastric polyps, Menetrier disease, partial gastrectomy, pernicious anemia, achlorhydria and hypochlorhydria represent risk conditions and may predispose to the development of adenocarcinoma of the stomach.

In 30% of cases gastric carcinoma is located on antrum, in 30% on gastric body and in other 30% on fundus or cardia; the remaining 10% is represented by diffuse infiltrating gastric lesions which affect all gastric walls at the time of diagnosis (Ba-Ssalamah et al, 2003).

Macroscopically, superficial forms, also called early gastric cancer, and advanced forms can be identified. Early gastric cancer is limited to the mucosal or submucosal layers and is characterized by variable incidence values from between 30% in Japan and 2 - 6% in other countries. Early gastric cancer can be difficult to recognize and can appear as a small, circumscribed, sometimes ulcerated thickening of the gastric wall (Angelelli et al, 2001).

The advanced gastric carcinoma reaches the muscolaris propria and four different kinds can be identified: polypoid, ulcerating, ulcerating-infiltrating and infiltrating forms, also called linitis plastica. Generally, in case of advanced gastric carcinoma, wall thickening exceeds 1 centimeter, with a variable extension, or a vegetating mass with irregular surfaces and a wide retracted base due to the invasion of the adjacent gastric wall can be identified.

The Jarvi and Lauren classification usually identifies intestinal or diffuse histological forms, the latest representing about the 80-90% of all gastric forms. The remaining 10-20% are represented by a third gastric form which collect all the other histological kinds. The intestinal form is usually moderately differentiated and originates from intestinal metaplasia areas; diffuse form represents an undifferentiated form which originated from gastric epithelium (Jarvi & Lauren, 1951).

In most of the cases gastric carcinoma has a preferential diffusion towards the cardia or it follows a contiguity, lymphatic or haematic mechanism. Usually, the intestinal form is less infiltrating, rarely can have a peritoneal involvement and can give hepatic metastatic nodules. On the contrary, diffuse gastric carcinoma rapidly involves adjacent structures and peritoneum.

However, metastatic diffusion usually depends on the extension and the depth of infiltration of the primary tumor. The most common metastatic sites are represented by lymph nodes (80% of cases), liver (40%), peritoneum (30%), lung (20%), pancreas (17%), retroperitoneum (12%), adrenal glands (10%), ovaries (5%) and diaphragm (5%).

Symptoms from gastric carcinoma are often non specific and also completely absent for a long time and tumor can be already advanced at the time of the diagnosis. Epigastric pain syndrome, dyspepsia, anemia, weight loss and weakness represent the most common symptoms.

Prognosis and therapy of gastric carcinoma depend on the stage of the disease at the time of the diagnosis and the first challenge for clinicians is to define the extent of the tumor in order to plan the best treatment (Kim JH et al, 2007; Moschetta et al, 2010).

Besides, an early diagnosis and accurate staging are crucial for the choice of an accurate therapeutic approach and can also influence the survival rate (Habermann et al, 2004). Surgery remains the main therapeutic option and the choice of the most suitable treatment is determined by preoperative staging, which is based on diagnostic imaging.

Radiation therapy or chemotherapy are reserved in selected cases.

2. Diagnostic imaging

Gastric carcinoma diagnosis usually bases on conventional barium radiological studies and endoscopy which often remain the first-line examination in the diagnostic approach to patients suspected of having gastric carcinoma. Both these techniques can identify initial mucosal lesions and endoscopy also allows to perform biopsies which are crucial for differentiating benign from malignant lesions, especially in case of ulcerative forms.

Transparietal ultrasound is often used in order to search for liver metastases and lymph node metastases (Stabile Ianora et al, 2001). Usually, the use of this tool complements computed tomography examination and could be useful in case of thin patients with low representation of fat planes.

Endoscopic ultrasound allows the identification of gastric wall stratification and the visualization of the different layers composing the gastric wall both in normal and pathological conditions. Diagnostic accuracy values from between 85% and 91% are

reported in literature for the evaluation of T parameter and from between 74% and 78% for N staging (Botet et al, 1991; Dittler & Siewert, 1993; Tunaci et al, 2002).
However, it represents an invasive and operator-dependent technique which does not allow the study of gastric walls below stenosing tumors or the visualization of distant lymphadenopathies or metastases (Ahn et al, 2009; Kwee et al, 2007; Moschetta et al, 2010).
The role of magnetic resonance imaging in the staging of gastric carcinoma is still unclear, but the use of this technique is increasing in this field, especially in case of pregnant women or in case of patients for whom uro-angiographic contrast agents are contraindicated. The reported accuracy values for magnetic resonance imaging range from 73% to 88% for T staging and from 55% to 65% for N staging (Arocena et al, 2006; Kim AY et al, 2000a, 2000b; Motohara et al, 2002; Sohn et al, 2000; Wang C-K et al, 2000). However, magnetic resonance imaging has some limitations, represented by longer examination time, motion artifacts and high cost.

3. Computed tomography

Computed tomography actually remains the most common and widespread tool for the staging of the disease and its reported accuracy values vary depending on the study technique and the device used (Moschetta et al, 2010; Stabile Ianora et al, 2001). In fact, computed tomography represents a valuable tool in addiction to gastroscopy and endoscopic ultrasound in the preoperative staging of gastric cancer.
It is the modality of choice for planning curative or palliative surgery and provides useful information for comparison during chemotherapy in patients with inoperable carcinomas (Yang et al, 2007).
The depth evaluation of gastric carcinoma mural invasion is improved with the clinical application of multidetector devices and multiplanar reconstructions. Therefore, multidetector computed tomography currently remains the most commonly used examination in the preoperative gastric cancer staging, with faster examination times and higher spatial resolution. In fact, it allows to acquire isotropic voxels and to reduce motion artifacts as compared to single-detector devices and the resulting benefits are represented by a better image quality in axial, coronal and sagittal planes and also better quality reconstructions, with an overall greater diagnostic accuracy.
Besides, the depth of tumor invasion has been shown to be a very important prognostic factor for these patients and the role of computed tomography is becoming stronger as technology improves, especially with bi-dimensional imaging (multi-planar reconstructions), tridimensional reconstructions (Volume Rendering) and virtual endoscopy (Blackshaw et al, 2005; Horton & Fishman, 2003; Moschetta et al, 2010).
The role of computed tomography in the study of gastric carcinoma is mainly represented by preoperative local and distant staging; post-therapeutic control and follow-up; incidental detection of gastric carcinoma during CT examination performed for other pathological conditions.

4. CT protocol

CT protocol is very important because it can affect the quality of CT examination.
First of all, before computed tomography examination, patients should be prepared by at least five hour fasting in order to empty the stomach.

Then, an adequate gastric distension is mandatory for the study of gastric walls; in fact, if stomach is not adequately distended, small gastric carcinomas can be misdiagnosed or collapsed gastric walls can simulate pathological conditions.
The gastric study on computed tomography examination needs therefore an adequate distension that can be obtained by using endoluminal contrast agents in order to distinguish gastric lumen and walls from adjacent structures and to allow an accurate evaluation of gastric wall thickness.
Gastrointestinal contrast agents can be subdivided in high density or positive and low density or negative agents, basing on the density values as compared with gastric walls. High density agents are mostly represented by diatrizoate and methyl-glucamine water solutions or barium solutions, the latest rarely used in this field.
Low density contrast agents are represented by water, air or CO2.
High density contrast agents are usually used in order to evaluate extra-gastric conditions, and in these cases gastric lumen and bowel loops are accurately delineated.
On the contrary, when a detailed study of gastric walls is required, it is better to avoid high density contrast agents because gastric walls present an increment of density after intravenous injection of contrast material in the site of lesion and small parietal lesions can be misdiagnosed because of the high density of gastric content. Occasionally, positive oral contrast agents may not mix uniformly with gastric contents and pseudotumors can be created.
Besides, also vascular or tridimensional studies can be difficult in case of high density agent's use. In fact, positive contrast agents can interfere with data manipulation during tri-dimensional imaging of the abdomen and necessitate extensive editing (Kim AY et al, 2005).
Therefore, in case of CT gastric carcinoma staging, the use of low density contrast material is preferred (Angelelli et al, 1987; Angelelli & Macarini, 1988; Moschetta et al, 2010; Rossi et al, 1997; Shimizu et al, 2005).
Among low density contrast materials, water represents a simple agent, with no cost or complication rate, well tolerated by patients and able to accurately distend the gastric cavity. Generally, a variable quantity from between 400 ml and 750 ml is ingested by patients ten minutes before CT examination, with a supplementary dose of 250 ml immediately before the scan.
Air also represents an accurate contrast agent for gastric evaluation on computed tomography, especially when virtual gastric endoscopy is planned in patients suspected of having gastric carcinoma. It can be administered as effervescent powders of bicarbonate or citric acid, which allow an optimal gastric distension.
Computed tomography examination also requires intravenous injection of iodinated contrast material which is mandatory to differentiate pathological tissue from normal mucosa and to obtain useful information for tumor characterization.
Usually, a quantity of 100-150 ml (mean value of 1.5 ml/kg body weight) is injected at 3-4 ml/sec.
The optimization of contrast material injection is essential in the era of multi-detector computed tomography, with higher time resolution. Although portal venous phase performed at 60-70 seconds from the intravenous injection is generally sufficient for a correct study of gastric walls, an additional arterial phase performed at 30-35 seconds from intravenous injection is useful for the staging of gastric primary lesions and for a better evaluation of the enhancement difference between gastric lesions and the adjacent normal tissue. Usually, the arterial phase is performed for upper abdomen while portal venous

phase includes thorax, abdomen and pelvis scanning, in order to perform distant staging of the disease.
Actually, bolus tracking and automated triggering technologies are generally used in order to obtain a correct biphasic technique basing on patient's characteristics.
Finally, in order to induce gastric wall hypotonia and decrease peristaltic bowel movement, 20 mg of scopolamine-N-butyl bromide can be intramuscularly or intravenously injected before CT examination.
CT scans are usually acquired in supine position; in rare cases, oblique patient position is recommended in order to evaluate some gastric portions, such as antrum or fundus (Moschetta et al, 2010; Shirakawa et al, 1996).

5. Image analysis

Computed tomography axial images and reconstructions are usually examined for diagnosis. Bi-dimensional multi-planar reconstructions on coronal and sagittal planes and tridimensional volume rendering reconstructions can be used in order to accurately diagnose and stage primary lesions (D'Elia et al, 2000) (Fig. 1).

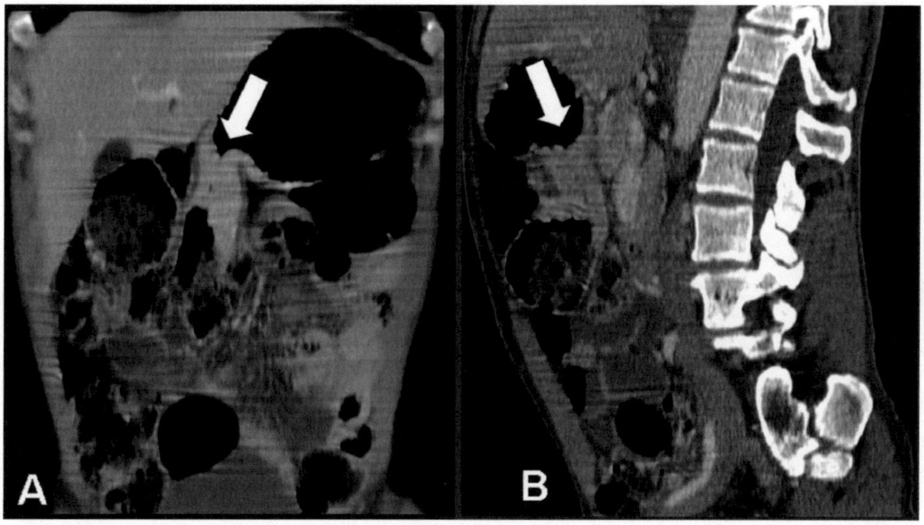

Fig. 1. Gastric carcinoma. A. CT Coronal Reconstruction. B. CT Sagittal Reconstruction. The tumor appears as an irregular wall thickening (arrows).

In case of air distension, virtual gastroscopy can be performed with endoluminal navigation and a direct visualization of gastric mucosal features (Fig. 2). Virtual endoscopy represents a tri-dimensional endoluminal-perspective image, which simulates the endoluminal views at gastroscopy. The detection of gastric cancer may be improved by multi-detector computed tomography with virtual gastroscopy (Bhandari et al, 2004; Kim HJ et al, 2005).
Besides, when ulcerative forms occur, virtual gastroscopy can also provide useful information for differentiating benign from malignant ulcers. In fact, benign ulcers usually present smooth and regular shapes, clearly demarcated and regular edges, with gastric fold tapering and converging toward the ulcer; on the contrary, in case of malignant ulcers, irregular shaped and asymmetric edges, disrupted appearance of peri-ulcer folds near the crater edge and fused folds can be identified.

On the other side, the use of a multiphasic technique after intravenous injection of contrast material allows to obtain an accurate imaging of gastric carcinoma and computed tomography can provide a complete dynamic visualization of the gastric walls in the site of carcinoma, enabling the calculation of whole-organ perfusion maps. In fact, computed tomography perfusion carries the potential to improve detection of gastric carcinoma due to the perfusion differences.

Recently, a new computed tomography reconstruction protocol called Vessel Probe in multi-planar mode has been shown to increase the diagnostic accuracy in T staging of gastric carcinoma in association with the water-filling technique for gastric distension (Moschetta et al, 2010).

The arterial phase is generally used to evaluate the T staging in these cases, in order to take advantage of the maximum enhancement of the gastric wall, which is essential to use vessel probe software.

Vessel Probe is a programme that allows vessels to be simultaneously examined in tri-dimensional, curved reformat and cross-sectional reformat views. It can study and measure arteries from between 0.5 and 18 mm in diameter and calculate the degree of stenosis. It can display images in a variety of formats, including automatic and simultaneous orthogonal cross-sections, orthogonal multi-planar, oblique and curved reconstructions, tri-dimensional and curved reformat views.

This fast and simple to use software can also be useful for examining the gastric wall on contrast-enhanced multi-detector computed tomography, clicking on the gastric wall in the lesion site. Starting from simple transverse images, Vessel Probe in multi-planar mode

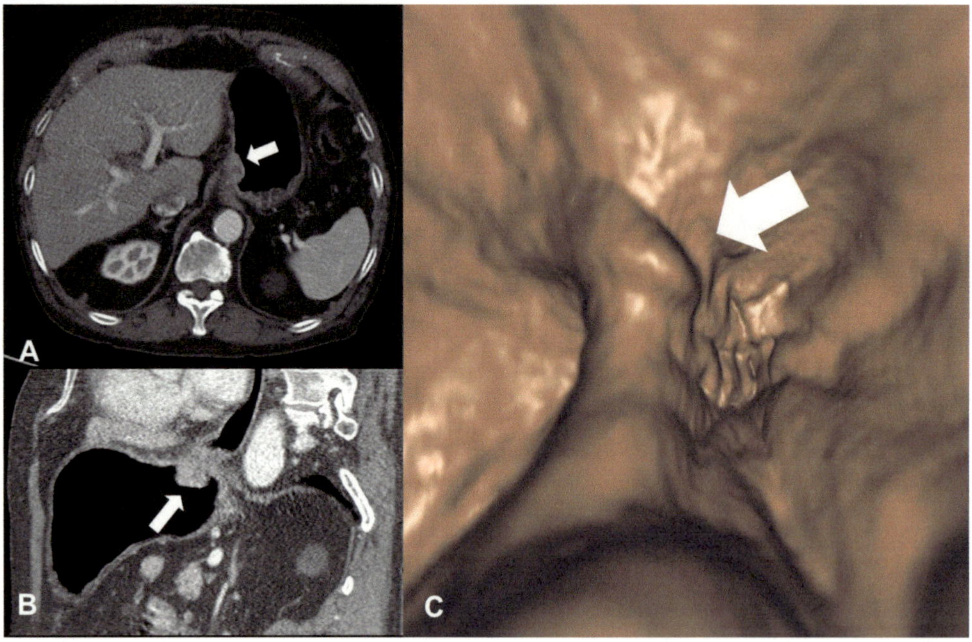

Fig. 2. Gastric carcinoma. A. CT transverse scan. B. CT multi-planar reconstruction on sagittal plane. C. Tri-dimensional virtual gastroscopy. The tumor appears as an irregular wall thickening protruding within gastric lumen and affecting the proximal tract of the stomach (arrows). Stomach has been distended by air.

automatically generates a reference line along the major axis of structures with the maximum enhancement values and displays the best views in multiple curved planes.
It also explores the whole thickness of the gastric wall and adjacent structures, which can be useful for T staging.

6. CT findings

Gastric carcinoma usually appears as an irregular wall thickening with high density after intravenous injection of contrast material, as compared with the contiguous normal gastric walls (Fig. 3). In the arterial phase, the neoplasm features a markedly greater density than the adjacent gastric walls, while in the venous phase this enhancement usually fades (Angelelli et al, 2001). More voluminous lesions can appear inhomogeneous because of the presence of necrotic areas.

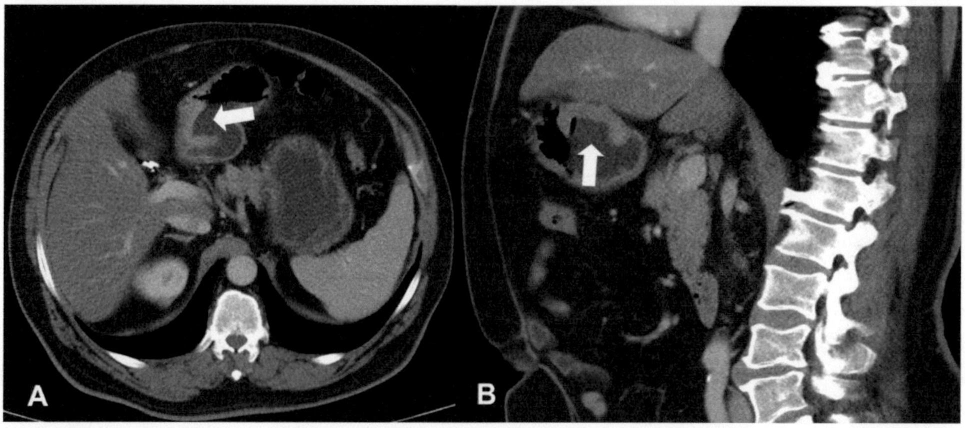

Fig. 3. Gastric carcinoma located on the antro-pyloric tract. A. CT transverse scan. B. CT reconstruction on sagittal plane. The tumor causes a focal area of irregular wall thickening with ulcerative features (arrows). Stomach has been distended by water.

Sometimes, during computed tomography examination of the abdomen performed for variable clinical or pathological conditions, gastric wall neoplastic thickenings can be incidentally detected.
Gastric carcinoma is generally subdivided in "early gastric cancer" and "advanced gastric cancer".
Early gastric cancer could have different forms:
Type I: lesion protruding more than 5 mm within gastric lumen;
Type IIa: lesion protruding less than 5 mm;
Type IIb: flat lesion;
Type IIc: concave lesion (not reaching muscularis mucosae);
Type III: ulcerative lesion (it reaches the muscolaris mucosae but not the muscolaris propria).
Multi-detector computed tomography examination allows to identify type I initial lesions while type II and III lesions can be more difficult to detect (Ba-Ssalamah et al, 2003). Sometimes, the histological characteristics can also influence the enhancement pattern of the primary lesion; in fact, it has been demonstrated that when a high mucin content is present,

the tumor can have low enhancement values also in the arterial phase and it can be very difficult to identify, especially when a thickening of gastric walls is not associated (Chen et al, 2007; Moschetta et al, 2010; Tunaci et al, 2002).

On the contrary, when adequate gastric distension is obtained, advanced cancer is usually easy to recognize at computed tomography examination and in 94% of cases it causes a circumscribed or diffuse wall thickening with associate ulcers or protruding lesions.

In case of linitis plastica, wall thickening is diffuse and circumferential with absence of the normal gastric folding. Besides, wall thickening can be variable and in some cases it can reach a diameter of some centimeters (Angelelli et al, 1990; Fukuya, 1997; Stabile Ianora et al, 2001).

In 6% of cases, tumor appears like a polypoid mass with a large implant base, or a vegetating lesion within gastric lumen and contiguous gastric walls can generally be thickened.

Neoplastic tissue usually presents low density values on computed tomography examination without contrast material injection as compared with normal gastric walls.

After intravenous injection of contrast medium, an increment of density values can be detected in most of the cases and rarely the tumor can appear isodense. The most voluminous tumors are inhomogeneous because of the presence of intralesional low density and colliquative areas. Rarely, some intralesional calcifications can also be detected.

Generally, a high density wall thickening should indicate gastric carcinoma; however, diagnosis should be always controlled by endoscopy and biopsy.

On the contrary, an isodense wall thickening is generally unspecific, and differential diagnosis with lymphomas, peptic ulcers, chronic gastritis, intestinal metaplasia, Zollinger-Ellison syndrome, amiloidosis, eosinophilic gastritis and Menetrier syndrome could be difficult in these cases.

In case of gastric carcinoma diagnosis, depth of intramural infiltration, extension towards contiguous structures and local and distant metastasis need to be evaluated.

Based on its appearance in the arterial phase, the gastric wall is defined as single-layered when only one high density layer can be visualised, or multi-layered when an inner high density and an outer low density layer can be identified.

T staging performed by computed tomography is crucial for the therapeutic approach to these patients and its precise diagnostic accuracy remains controversial (Kadowaki et al, 2000; Kumano S et al, 2005; Minami et al, 1997).

According to the TNM classification and computed tomography staging criteria, T1 tumors invade lamina propria or submucosal layer and can appear as circumscribed wall thickening with intense focal enhancement or intense enhancement only, without wall thickening or circumscribed wall thickening with intense enhancement of inner layer and a low density streak corresponding to the non infiltrated muscolaris propria coat on computed tomography examination.

T2 tumors invade the muscolaris propria or subserosa and appear as thickening of entire gastric wall with homogeneous or inhomogeneous enhancement, regular surface of the outer layer of gastric wall at the lesion site and normal appearance of perigastric fat.

T3 gastric carcinomas invade serosa without infiltration of adjacent structures and generally are represented by thickening of entire gastric wall with homogeneous or inhomogeneous enhancement, irregular surface of the outer layer of gastric wall at the lesion site and presence of micronodules or dense stranding in the perigastric fat on computed tomography examination.

Finally, T4 gastric tumors are characterized by the invasion of adjacent structures and the obliteration of the fat cleavage plane between the neoplastic lesion and adjacent organs.

Diagnostic accuracy values from between 41% and 98% have been reported in literature for the computed tomography evaluation of T parameter (Moschetta, 2010; Stabile Ianora, 2003); the controversy with regard to the effective role of this tool for the T staging of gastric cancer, especially in the evaluation of early gastric cancer, probably bases on the different used technique. In fact, the increasing values reported in recent studies are probably due to the high quality of multi-planar images produced by using a thin-slice collimation, isotropic voxels and better z-axis resolution.

As already reported before, some interesting new data emerge with regard to the differentiation between various T stages by using the Vessel Probe reconstructions (Moschetta et al, 2010).

This programme allows good detail of the gastric wall architecture to be obtained after the intravenous injection of contrast material and it can improve the diagnostic accuracy in the evaluation of the tumor invasion depth by analysing the wall enhancement in the lesion site. Generally, images obtained during the arterial phase are useful for the application of the Vessel Probe in the T staging because of the tumor hypervascularity and neovascularity (Lee JH et al, 2007; Moschetta et al, 2010). In fact, by using the tumor enhancement, the Vessel Probe algorithm permits a more accurate view of the gastric wall stratification as compared with the other computed tomography reconstructions. The high quality of these new reconstructions can also help to solve the problem of the differentiation between T2 and T3 gastric carcinoma. In fact, the reticular and dense stranding in the perilesional fat and the irregular appearance of the outer surface of the gastric walls can usually identify T3 carcinomas, but can also be seen in inflammatory reactions without cancer infiltration (Chen et al, 2006; Takao et al, 1998).

Vessel Probe reformatting images reduce partial volume artifacts and improve the evaluation of the gastric wall surface in orthogonal views.

Besides, the high spatial resolution may be helpful when the fat cleavage plane between the tumor and the adjacent organs is oblique or parallel to the imaging direction.

Finally, this kind of automatic post-processing can be obtained in a few minutes per patient and is therefore faster than tri-dimensional imaging of the gastric cancer, especially with regard to virtual gastroscopy; compared with simple multi-planar reconstructions, Vessel Probe algorithm allows the best view of gastric wall stratification to be automatically displayed in the lesion site, by simultaneously reconstructing images in multiplanar, perpendicular curved and oblique planar reformats (Fig. 4).

Gastric tumor located on the proximal part of the stomach can involve peritoneum, left liver lobe, diaphragm, spleen and aorta; tumors located on the distal tract can also involve the pancreas.

The main criteria for the diagnosis of tumor diffusion towards contiguous structures are based on the evaluation of perigastric fat tissue which can be preserved or infiltrated by high density stranding. However, in patients with poor nutritional conditions with a low representation of fat tissue, it could be difficult to evaluate the anatomical relationships of a tumor located on the posterior gastric surface with adjacent structures, such as pancreas. Besides, as reported before, the irregular extern gastric surface or the presence of dense tissue within the perigastric fat tissue could sometimes be determined by desmoplastic or inflammatory reactions. In these cases, overstaging can occur.

Some experiences also reported that a neoplastic involvement of adjacent organs was present, although a clear perigastric adipose clivage was identifiable, thus determining understaging mistakes.

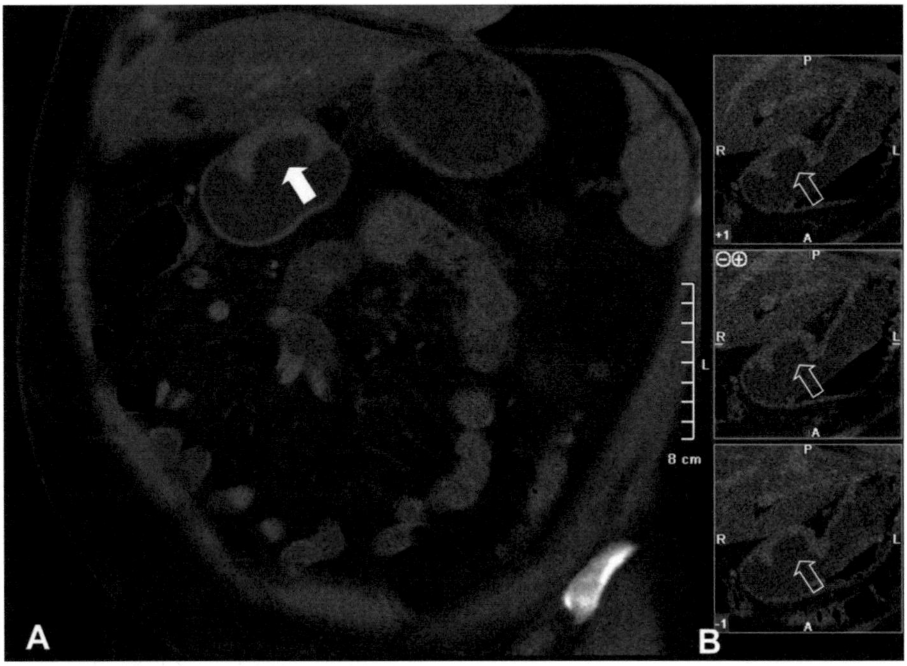

Fig. 4. Gastric ulcerative carcinoma. Same patient as in Fig. 3. A. CT reconstruction on oblique coronal plane. The tumor appears as an ulcerating wall thickening (arrow). B. Vessel Probe reconstructions allow to obtain a better identification of the gastric wall in the lesion site (empty arrows).

Sometimes, gastric carcinoma can also involve the mesocolon or gastro-splenic, gastro-hepatic and hepato-duodenal ligaments through the sierosa.

The identification of peritoneal involvement could be very difficult on computed tomography and often it can be possible only in advanced forms. Ascites and peritoneal nodules, mostly located on the mesocolon, represent the most common signs in these cases.

Lymph nodal involvement is generally recognized in 74 - 88% of patients with gastric carcinoma because of a wide perigastric net of lymphatic drain and its incidence can be related to tumor size and depth of infiltration. N staging need to involve all 16 nodal perigastric stations and it is recommended to distinguish between the involvement of perigastric nodal sites, with a distance of less then 3 cm from the organ, and extragastric nodal sites, for example following the left gastric artery, the common hepatic artery, the splenic artery or the celiac trunk, or distant nodal metastases, for example at the hepato-duodenal ligament, retropancreatic, mesenteric or para-aortic sites (Fig. 5). In fact, all gastric carcinomas with involvement of perigastric lymph nodes located at less than 3 cm away from the primary lesion are classified as N1; those with involvement of extragastric lymph nodes located at more than 3 cm away from the primary lesion as N2; finally, N3 forms involve lymph nodes of retroperitoneum or the hepatic-duodenal ligament.

Because of the panoramic view and anatomical detail, computed tomography represents a fundamental examination for recognizing locoregional, perigastric and distant adenopathies.

However, computed tomography evaluation of N parameter is still actually challenging and still has several limitations in this field, with a reported accuracy value of 70%. In fact,

computed tomography is not able to identify neoplastic lymph nodes with normal size (false negatives) or it can not differentiate larger reactive lymph nodes (false positives).
In order to reduce the number of false positives, number and enhancement values of lymph nodes could be also considered. The presence of numerous lymphadenopathies suggest a metastatic disease in 96% of cases while a single larger lymph node in 48% of cases. Metastatic lymph nodes are often characterized by different enhancement values as compared with normal nodes.
Other difficulties in this field can be represented by the site of lymph nodes, the morphology of the tumor and the patient characteristics. In fact, in case of voluminous tumors with a prevalent extragastric development it can be difficult to detect lymph nodes strictly adherent to the gastric walls.
Moreover, some nodal sites are more difficult to explore, such as paracardial or hepato-duodenal sites.
Finally, patient's characteristics are also important because, in case of cachectic subjects with poor adipose representation, it can be more difficult to recognize lymphadenopaties.
Therefore, computed tomography is relatively insensitive and also non specific for detecting nodal metastases because of its inability to recognize microscopic nodal invasion, which is common in gastric carcinoma, and the presence of reactive lymph nodes that may have increased size. Multi-planar reconstruction seem slightly better than transverse images for N staging (Chen et al, 2007). In fact, they can provide more accurate measurement of lymph node size and better differentiation between lymph nodes and small perigastric vessels (Fig. 6).
Thus, it is recommended to indicate all visible lymph nodes, independently from diameter and indicating histology for definitive diagnosis and an accurate N staging.

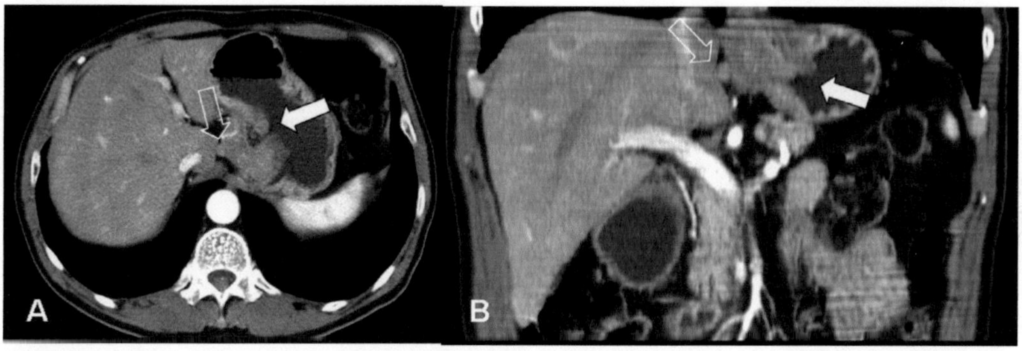

Fig. 5. A. CT Transverse Scan. B. CT Coronal Reconstruction. Gastric carcinoma causes an irregular wall thickening on the proximal tract of the stomach (arrows). Peri-gastric suspected lymph nodes are associated (empty arrows).

In planning treatment, it is essential to define the presence of any secondary localization of the disease. The staging of M parameter includes M0 stage, in case of absence of distant metastases and M1 stage, in case of presence of distant metastases. Haematic metastases more often involve the liver, because gastric venous drain is mostly performed by portal circle; less commonly, lungs, adrenal glands, kidneys, bone and brain can be involved. In advanced forms, peritoneal involvement occurs for contiguity and in women it can also cause ovarian metastases (Krukenberg tumors).
The diagnostic accuracy of computed tomography for the evaluation of the M parameter reaches 97% and 100% (Stabile Ianora et al, 2003).

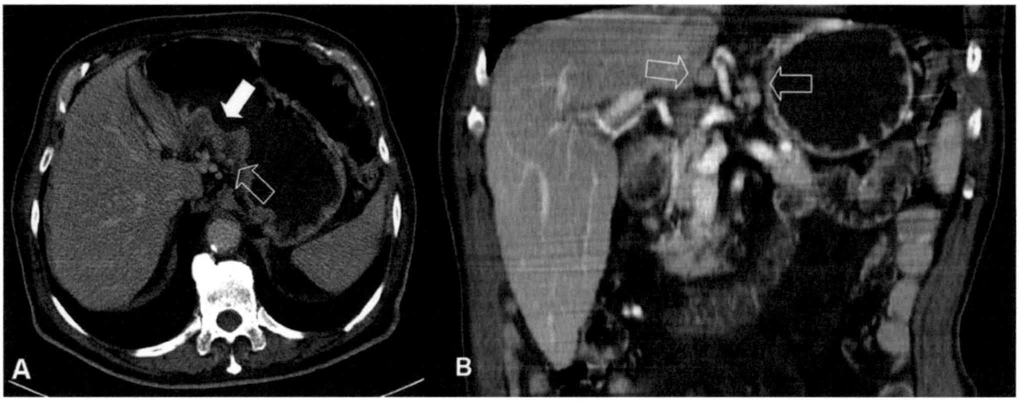

Fig. 6. A. CT Transverse Scan. B. CT Coronal Reconstruction. The tumoral tissue is well evident (arrow). Several suspected peri-gastric lymph nodes are associated (empty arrows).

7. Post-therapy control

In the past, traditional radiological studies were used in surgically treated patients with the possibility of providing morphological and functional information on the anastomosis and identifying mucosal lesions. These techniques are actually reserved to selected cases and widely replaced in clinical practice by endoscopy which allows a direct visualization of gastric mucosa with the possibility of performing biopsies in suspected areas.
Computed tomography imaging also represents an accurate technique in this field, because it allows to evaluate the anatomical relationships after surgical treatment and also the presence of complications, such as anastomosis dehiscence, hemorrhage or abscesses.
Neoplastic relapse such as extramural tumor or gastric stump carcinoma and distant metastases can be easily detected at follow-up performed by computed tomography examinations.
Gastric stump carcinoma is defined as primary tumor arising from the gastric stump, usually 15-20 years later partial gastrectomy.
Generally, the affected patients underwent gastro-jejunumstomy (Billroth II) rather than gastro-duodenostomy (Billroth I). These tumors are usually located on the distal tract of gastric stump, close to the anastomosis (Ba-Ssalamah et al, 2003).
A pathogenetic theory related to a biliary reflux above the anastomosis with consequent chronic gastritis and metaplasia has been proposed in these cases. Gastric stump carcinoma and neoplastic recurrences are detected on computed tomography as wall thickenings or small masses close to the anastomosis.
However, not all peri-anastomotic thickenings are caused by neoplastic recurrence, because they can be determined by surgical folds, bowel adhesions or polypoid hypertrophic gastritis.
An adequate technique and the use of multi-planar and tri-dimensional reconstructions with the possibility of virtual navigation within the lumen allow to increase diagnostic accuracy values, but in suspected cases it is mandatory an endoscopic and histological control (Quarticelli et al, 2004).
The contribution of computed tomography is also reliable in case of patients subjected to chemo-radiotherapy in order to evaluate the response to the therapy, although when

residual masses are detected, it can be difficult to differentiate the neoplastic or fibrotic nature of these lesions.

8. Conclusions

Computed tomography represents an accurate tool in case of gastric carcinoma. It is important to associate the axial image examination with the analysis of multi-planar, Vessel Probe and tri-dimensional reconstructions.

Multi-planar images are widely used; they increase diagnostic accuracy for the evaluation of the tumor extension, the anatomical relationships with contiguous organs and facilitate the identification of lymph nodal and distant metastases.

Vessel Probe reconstructions can facilitate T staging of gastric carcinoma, especially in the arterial phase of computed tomography examination.

Tri-dimensional reconstructions provide a volumetric evaluation of the gastric walls, with consequent diagnostic advantages in modifying the transparency levels and detecting vascular structures or gastric walls.

Virtual gastroscopy is also accurate in detecting gastric lesions, with the possibility of information which well correlate with traditional endoscopy findings.

9. References

Ahn HS, Lee HJ, Yoo MW, Kim SG, Im JP, Kim SH, Kim WH, Lee KU & Yang HK (2009). Diagnostic accuracy of T and N stages with endoscopy, stomach protocol CT, and endoscopic ultrasonography in early gastric cancer. *J Surg Oncol* 99: 20-27.

Angelelli G & Macarini L (1988). CT of the bowel: use of water to enhance depiction. *Radiology* 169:848-9.

Angelelli G, Macarini L & Favia G (1990). The CT aspects and pathological correlations in gastric adenocarcinoma and lymphoma. *Radiol Med* 79:191-6.

Angelelli G, Macarini L & Fratello A (1987). Use of water as an oral contrast agent for CT study of the stomach. *AJR Am J Roentgenol* 149:1084.

Angelelli G, Stabile Ianora AA, Scardapane A, Pedote P, Memeo M & Rotondo A (2001). Role of computerized tomography in the staging of gastrointestinal neoplasm. *Semin Surg Oncol* 20:109-121.

Arocena MG, Barturen A, Bujanda L, Casado O, Ramírez MM, Oleagoitia JM, Galdiz Iturri M, Múgica P, Cosme A, Gutiérrez-Stampa MA, Zapata E & Echenique-Elizondo M (2006). MRI and endoscopic ultrasonography in the staging of gastric cancer. *Rev Esp Enferm Dig* 98: 582-590.

Ba-Ssalamah A, Prokop M, Uffmann M, Pokieser P, Teleky B & Lechner G (2003). Dedicated multidetector CT of the stomach: spectrum of diseases. *Radiographics* 23:625-44.

Bhandari S, Shim CS, Kim JH, Jung IS, Cho JY, Lee JS, Lee MS & Kim BS (2004). Usefulness of three-dimensional, multidetector row CT (virtual gastroscopy and multiplanar reconstruction) in the evaluation of gastric cancer: a comparison with conventional endoscopy, EUS and histopathology. *Gastrointest Endosc* 59: 619-626.

Blackshaw GR, Stephens MR, Lewis WG, Boyce J, Barry JD, Edwards P, Allison MC & Thomas GV (2005). Progressive CT system technology and experience improve the perceived preoperative stage of gastric cancer. *Gastric Cancer* 8: 29-34.

Botet JF, Lightdale CJ, Zauber AG, Gerdes H, Winawer SJ, Urmacher C & Brennan MF (1991). Preoperative staging of gastric carcinoma: comparison of endoscopic US and dynamic CT. *Radiology* 181: 426-432.

Chen CY, Hsu JS, Wu DC, Kang WY, Hsieh JS, Jaw TS, Wu MT & Liu GC (2007). Gastric cancer: preoperative local staging with 3D multi-detector row CT - correlation with surgical and histopathologic results. *Radiology* 242: 472-482.

Chen CY, Wu DC, Kang WY & Hsu JS (2006). Staging of gastric cancer with 16-channel MDCT. *Abdom Imaging* 31: 514-520.

D'Elia F, Zingarelli A, Palli D & Grani M (2000). Hydro-dynamic CT preoperative staging of gastric cancer: correlation with pathological findings. A prospective study of 107 cases. *Eur Radiol* 10:1877-1885.

Dittler HJ & Siewert JR (1993). Role of endoscopic ultrasonography in gastric carcinoma. *Endoscopy* 25: 162-6.

Fishman EK, Urban BA & Hruban RH (1996). CT of the stomach: spectrum of disease. *Radiographics* 16:1035-54.

Fukuya T, Honda H, Kaneko K, Kuroiwa T, Yoshimitsu K, Irie H, Maehara Y & Masuda K (1997). Efficacy of helical CT in T staging of gastric cancer. *J Comput Assist Tomogr* 21: 73-81.

Habermann CR, Weiss F, Riecken R, Honarpisheh H, Bohnacker S, Staedtler C, Dieckmann C, Schoder V & Adam G (2004). Preoperative staging of gastric adenocarcinoma: comparison of helical CT and endoscopic US. *Radiology* 230: 465-71.

Horton KM & Fishman EK (2003). Current role of CT in imaging of the stomach. *Radiographics* 23:75-87.

Jarvi O & Lauren P (1951). On the role of heterotopias of the intestinal epithelium in the pathogenesis of gastric cancer. *Acta Pathol Microbiol Scand* 29:26-44.

Kadowaki K, Murakami T, Yoshioka H, Kim T, Takahashi S, Tomoda K, Narumi Y & Nakamura H (2000). Helical CT imaging of gastric cancer: normal wall appearance and the potential for staging. *Radiat Med* 18: 47-54.

Kim AY, Han JK, Kim TK, Park SJ & Choi BI (2000). MR imaging of advanced gastric cancer: comparison of various MR pulse sequences using water and gadopentetate dimeglumine as oral contrast agents. *Abdom Imaging* 25: 7-13.

Kim AY, Han JK, Seong CK, Kim TK & Choi BI (2000). MRI in staging advanced cancer: is it useful compared with spiral CT? *J Comput Assist Tomogr* 24:389-94.

Kim AY, Kim HJ & Ha HK. (2005) Gastric cancer by multidetector row CT: preoperative staging. *Abdom Imaging* 30: 465-472.

Kim HJ, Kim AY, Oh ST, Kim JS, Kim KW, Kim PN, Lee MG & Ha HK (2005). Gastric cancer staging at multi-detector row CT gastrography: comparison of transverse and volumetric CT scanning. *Radiology* 236: 879-885.

Kim JH, Eun HW, Choi JH, Hong SS, Kang W & Auh YH (2007). Diagnostic performance of virtual gastroscopy using MDCT in early gastric cancer compared with 2D axial CT: focusing on interobserver variation. *Am J Roentgenol* 189: 299-305.

Kim JH, Eun HW, Goo DE, Shim CS & Auh YH (2006). Imaging of various gastric lesions with 2D MPR and CT gastrography performed with multidetector CT. *Radiographics* 26:1101-16.

Kumano S, Murakami T, Kim T, Hori M, Iannaccone R, Nakata S, Onishi H, Osuga K, Tomoda K, Catalano C & Nakamura H (2005). T staging of gastric cancer: role of multi-detector row CT. *Radiology* 237: 961-966.

Kwee RM & Kwee TC. (2007) Imaging in local staging of gastric cancer: a systematic review. *J Clin Oncol* 25: 2107-2116.

Lee DH (2000). Two-dimensional and three-dimensional imaging of gastric tumors using spiral CT. *Abdom Imaging* 25: 1-6.

Lee JH, Jeong YK, Kim DH, Go BK, Woo YJ, Ham SY & Yang SO (2007). Two-phase helical CT for detection of early gastric carcinoma: importance of the mucosal phase for analysis of the abnormal mucosal layer. *J Comput Assist Tomogr* 24: 777-782.

Levine MS & Megibow AJ (1994). Gastric carcinoma. In: Gore RM, Levine MS, Laufer I, Eds. *Textbook of gastrointestinal radiology*. Philadelphia, Pa: Saunders, pp. 600-83.

Minami M, Kawauchi N, Itai Y, Niki T & Sasaki Y. (1992) Gastric tumors: radiologic-pathologic correlation and accuracy of T staging with dynamic CT. *Radiology* 185: 173-178.

Moschetta M, Stabile Ianora AA, Anglani A, Marzullo A, Scardapane A & Angelelli G (2010). Preoperative T staging of gastric carcinoma obtained by MDCT vessel probe reconstructions and correlations with histological findings. *Eur Radiol.* 20:138-45.

Motohara T & Semelka RC. (2002) MRI in staging of gastric cancer. *Abdom Imaging* 27: 376-383.

Quarticelli T, Scardapane A, Memeo M, Calbi R, Stabile Ianora AA & Angelelli G (2004). Multidetector CT assessment of postgastrectomy patients. *Radiol Med* 107:317-24.

Rossi M, Broglia L, Arata FM, Di Girolamo M, Petrone A, Coniglio M & Rossi P (1997). The diagnostic accuracy and reproducibility of computed tomography with water distention and induced hypotonia in the preoperative staging of gastric tumors. *Radiol Med* 94: 486-491.

Shimizu K, Ito K, Matsunaga N, Shimizu A & Kawakami Y (2005). Diagnosis of gastric cancer with MDCT using the water-filling method and multiplanar reconstruction: CT-histologic correlation. *Am J Roentgenol* 185:1152-1158.

Shirakawa T, Fukuda K & Tada S. (1996) New method for evaluation of perigastric invasion of gastric cancer by right lateral position CT. *Eur Radiol* 6: 358-361.

Sohn KM, Lee JM, Lee SY, Ahn BY, Park SM & Kim KM (2000). Comparing MR imaging and CT in the staging of gastric carcinoma. *Am J Roentgenol* 174: 1551-1557.

Stabile Ianora AA, Pedote P, Scardapane A, Memeo M, Rotondo A & Angelelli G (2003). Preoperative staging of gastric carcinoma with multi detector spiral CT. *Radiol Med* 106: 467-480.

Stabile Ianora AA, Wolowiec A, Francioso G, Scardapane A, Rotondo A & Angelelli G (2001). Benign and malignant gastric ulcer: CT findings. *Radiol Med* 102: 32-36.

Takao M, Fukuda T, Iwanaga S, Hayashi K, Kusano H & Okudaira S (1998). Gastric cancer: evaluation of triphasic spiral CT and radiologic-pathological correlation. *J Comput Assist Tomogr* 22: 288-294.

Tunaci M (2002). Carcinoma of stomach and duodenum: radiologic diagnosis and staging. *Eur J Radiol* 42: 181-192.

Wang C-K, Kuo Y-T, Liu G-C, Tsai KB & Huang YS (2000). Dynamic contrast-enhanced subtraction and delayed MRI of gastric tumours: radiologic-pathological correlation. *J Comput Assist Tomogr* 24: 872-7.

Yang DM, Kim HC, Jin W, Ryu CW, Kang JH, Park CH, Kim HS & Jung DH (2007). 64 multidetector-row computed tomography for preoperative evaluation of gastric cancer: histological correlation. *J Comput Assist Tomogr* 31: 98-103.

2

MR Imaging of Gastric Carcinoma

Il Young Kim
Soonchunhyang University
Republic of Korea

1. Introduction

Magnetic Resonance (MR) imaging has not become popular for staging of gastric carcinoma because of a number of limitations, including motion artifacts, lack of a stable contrast medium, and the high cost. However, continuous technical improvements have been made in MR imaging of the abdomen, thereby reducing motion artifacts and improving image quality. These improvements include breath-hold fast imaging techniques, placement of abdominal binders, administration of antiperistaltic agents, and the use of phased array coils. In vitro studies using 1 - 4.7- T MR systems have shown that MRI allows the depiction of gastric wall layers and therefore, technically permits the evaluation of the local tumor stage of gastric carcinomas. However, MR study in gastric carcinoma is challenging and it has much possibility. Usually, the preoperative staging workup of gastric carcinoma is performed mainly with computed tomography (CT). CT has been a favored method for preoperative evaluation and staging in patients with gastric carcinoma (Goldberg & Thoeni. 1989; Werthmuller & Margulis. 1991; Halvorsen & Thompson. 1991). Parallel advances in CT equipment and scanning techniques have reduced scanning time and decreased motion artifacts. Simultaneously, rapid IV contrast administration with an automatic power injector has improved contrast enhancement of the gastric wall and gastric carcinoma. Helical CT has advantages over conventional CT, including faster scanning time and fewer respiratory misregistration artifacts in a single breath-hold (Hahn, et al., as cited in Stark & Bradley. 1992). However, CT is limited, particularly in the diagnosis of lymph node metastasis, peritoneal metastasis, and small hematogenous metastasis. Endoscopic sonography has been reported to be the most accurate technique for the T staging of gastric carcinoma because it can define five layers of the gastric wall (Botet, et al. 1991). But this technique cannot evaluate other factors such as liver metastasis and peritoneal seeding. In addition, endoscopic sonography is an invasive technique dependent on the operator.

2. MR Imaging

2.1 MR Imaging techniques

Residual stool or foodstuff can obviate the evaluation of gastrointestinal wall structures. Therefore, MRI should be performed following a 6 hr fasting period to ensure a consistent assessment of the stomach. A reliable distension of stomach must be achieved to allow for a reliable evaluation of the gastric wall. Otherwise, insufficient distension may result in false-positive or false-negative findings. Adequate distension of the stomach can be easily accomplished by oral administration of water or water based contrast agents. Image data should be collected without any time delay after contrast administration. Fast breath-hold MR sequences and antiperistaltic drugs are suggested for gastric carcinoma patient. A large volume (1 L) of tap water is ingested to the patient for the distention and opacification of the stomach (Seong, et al. 1998). This large volume of water was tolerated by the patients while providing sufficient distention of the stomach, which made it easier to differentiate gastric carcinoma from normal gastric wall. Water is absolutely safe and does not cause susceptibility artifacts. Sohn et al. (2000) used water or effervescent granules as oral contrast agents. Water is biphasic and the simplest contrast agent. Effervescent granules (a negative contrast agent) make the lumen of the stomach dark. If the stomach is overly distended with air, a magnetic susceptibility artifact may occur. However, the use of effervescent granules still provides improved evaluation of the gastric wall and can be used to supplement or replace water for gastric distention (Halvorsen, et al. 1996). Furthermore, oral Gd-DTPA does not provide additional diagnostic information over using tap water in MRI for gastric carcinoma (Kim A., et al. 2000a, 2000b). Therefore, the water-filling method may be appropriate for MRI of advanced gastric carcinoma (AGC).

There are various techniques for performing MR scanning. Sohn et al. (2000) used that imaging technique with a superconductive magnet operating at 1.5 T with a phased array coil. Patients fasted for 6 hr and ingested 500ml of water or effervescent granules as an oral contrast agent. Twenty milligrams of scopolamine (Buscopan; Boehringer International, Ingelheim, Germany) were administered intramuscularly 5 min before the examination for decrease of bowel peristalsis. Patients can be placed on the MR gantry in the supine or prone position to allow the lesion to contact the ingested water or air. When water was used as the oral contrast agent, the patients in whom the lesion was at the gastric cardia or fundus were imaged in the supine position, and the other patients were imaged in the prone position. The positions were reversed when effervescent granules were used as or patients were examined with a breath-hold T1-weighted 2D FLASH technique in the axial, coronal, and sagittal planes. The scanning parameters for T1-weighted axial images were TR/TE, 146.1/4.1 msec; flip angle, 80°; and one excitation. The bandwidth was 260 Hz; field of view, 33 cm; matrix size, 128× 256; and the slice thickness was 8 mm with a 1.6-mm gap. The scan time was 18 sec. The parameters for the T1-weighted coronal and sagittal images were the same as those for T1-weighted axial images, except for the TR (100 for coronal and sagittal images) and field of view (45 cm for coronal images). The scan times of coronal and sagittal images were 14 and 12 sec, respectively. T2-weighted axial turbo spin-echo images were obtained with a TR/TE of 3200/138, an echo spacing of 9.2 msec, an echo train length of 29, a flip angle of 18°, one excitation, a bandwidth of 260 Hz, a field of view of 33 cm, a matrix size of 116 × 256, an 8-mm slice thickness with a gap of 1.6 mm, and a scan time of 17 sec. Sixty seconds after an IV bolus injection of 15–20 mg of gadopentetate dimeglumine (Magnevist; Schering, Berlin, Germany) at a rate of approximately 1 ml/sec through an antecubital vein, axial T1-weighted FLASH images with fat suppression were obtained (157.6/4.1; flip angle, 80°; one excitation; bandwidth, 260 Hz; field of view, 33 cm; matrix size, 128× 256; slice thickness, 8 mm; gap, 1.6 mm) with a scan time of 19 sec. All sequences were performed in a single breath-hold. Nineteen slices were obtained for unenhanced and contrast-enhanced T1-weighted axial images, and 11 slices were obtained for coronal and sagittal T1- and T2-weighted images. For fast MR imaging, Sohn et al. (2000) performed breathhold T1-weighted 2D FLASH, T2-weighted turbo spin-echo, and contrast-enhanced T1- weighted FLASH sequences with fat suppression. In most cases, Sohn et al. (2000)

staged the tumor with two or three planes (axial, coronal, and sagittal) of unenhanced T1-weighted images only. Sohn et al. (2000) used the fat suppression technique in contrast-enhanced MR imaging to make the contrast between enhanced gastric tumor and perigastric fat more conspicuous. However, contrast-enhanced T1-weighted images showed more artifacts and lower visual contrast than unenhanced T1-weighted images. The T2- weighted images showed little difference in signal intensity between tumor and normal gastric wall and did not show an advantage for tissue characterization. Coronal and sagittal images were useful for evaluation of extraluminal outgrowth and omental infiltration by tumor. MR images, even with breath-hold fast MR imaging, were not completely free from motion artifacts, and sometimes a ghost artifact from aortic pulsation hid a lesion at the gastric angle.

On the other study, Kim A et al. (2000) used a 1.0 T scanner with a body phased array coil. Axial, coronal, and sagittal images of fast low angle shot (FLASH; TR/TE 160/6.6 ms, flip angle 75°, one excitation, matrix size 256 × 112), half-Fourier single shot turbo SE (HASTE; infinite TR, echo space 10.9 ms, TE 87 ms, flip angle 150°, matrix size 256 × 240), and true fast imaging with steady-state precession (true-FISP; TR/TE 7.6/3.5 ms, one excitation, flip angle 80°, matrix size 256 × 192) sequences were obtained in each patient immediately after ingestion of 1 L of tap water. Field of view varied from 40 to 42 cm. In all MR pulse sequences, 8 mm thickness scans were obtained during a single breath-hold. In each patient, spiral CT or MRI was performed after overnight fasting to empty the stomach. Time interval between the two examinations was either 1 or 2 days. Twenty milligrams of scopolamine (Buscopan; Boehringer International, Ingelheim, Germany) was given intramuscularly to reduce peristaltic bowel movement before MR examinations. Except for one patient in whom the lesion was located in the gastric fundus and who had images taken in the supine position, all other patients were imaged in the prone position.

2.2 MR imaging protocol of resected stomach

There is MR imaging study with gastric specimen by Kim I et al. (2009). In this study, there is gastric specimen distention with filling of saline solution. 1.5-T MRI is used for this study with the following multisection spin echo sequences for T1-weighted images, repetition time (TR) m sec/echo time (TE) m sec = 500/20, and for T2-weighted images, 2500/90. Two numbers of excitation were applied in this scanning. The matrix size was 256X 256. Slice thickness was 5 mm and the intersection gap was 1 mm. Field of view was 20 cm. MR scans of the gastrectomy specimen were taken along the axial and sagittal planes. A head coil was used for scanning.

2.3.1 Image analysis of gastric carcinoma

A lesion is considered a cancerous lesion when the thickness of the gastric wall is >6mm and abrupt transition is noted between the thickened and adjacent normal gastric wall (Matsushita, et al. 1994). A lymph node of >8 mm on its short axis is considered to be pathologic (Dorfman, et al. 1991). The depth of tumor invasion on MRI is determined as follows: mT1 (no abnormal findings), mT2 (a clear and smooth outer surface of the lesion on FLASH/HASTE or intact low signal intensity band surrounding the lesion on true-FISP), mT3 (an irregular outer surface with obliteration of perigastric fat plane on FLASH/HASTE or interrupted low signal intensity band around the lesion on true-FISP), and mT4 (contiguous extension of gastric lesion to adjacent organs on any pulse sequences).

2.3.2 Image analysis of resected stomach

The number of visible wall layers and their specific signal intensity (SI) characteristics are studied by Kim I et al. (2009). Wall-layer correlation was made on the basis of the layer thickness of the visible layers in MRI compared with the ones visible in histology. The presence of a tumor, defined as destruction of the normal gastric wall layers, is noted. The tumors are examined for variations in SI. The depth of infiltration is evaluated according to earlier publications (Dux M., et al. 1997; Cho J-S., et al. 1994). A normal gastric wall is identified as having 3 layers. In terms of scanning direction and degree of distention of the wall, a gastric wall that is more than 1 cm thick or that showed an abrupt change of pattern from normal to pathologic is considered abnormal. The location, gross appearance, size and degree of serosal invasion of tumors are evaluated. Location is classified according to four areas: antrum, body, body and antrum, and fundus. Gross appearance is classified into four categories by Bormann's classification for advanced gastric carcinoma (Douglass, Nava. 1985). T and N staging were based on the TNM system developed by the American Joint Committee on Cancer (AJCC. 2002). Early gastric cancer is evaluated according to the Japanese Research Society for Gastric Cancer (Kajitani. 1981). The degree of tumor invasion in the gastric wall according to the T stage is measured as follows: T1 meant that MR showed obliteration of SI within the thickened mucosal layer and second submucosal layer, T2 meant that thickening of the gastric wall and obliteration of the third layer of muscularis propria, and T3 meant irregular SI in the outer margin of the third layer.

The total number of lymph nodes which were located in the perigastric area is counted. A lymph node of >8mm at the short axis is considered to be pathologic (Dorfman, et al. 1991). N staging of lymph nodes was performed. N0 is defined as no regional lymph node metastasis, N1 as metastasis in one to six regional lymph nodes, N2 as metastasis in seven to 15 regional lymph nodes, N3 as metastasis in more than 15 regional lymph nodes.

3. MR imaging finding of gastric carcinoma

3.1 T staging of gastric carcinoma

CT is widely used as a primary imaging modality for preoperative staging of gastric cancer. Although CT provides detailed information regarding the extent of tumor spread and provides guidelines to surgeons to avoid unnecessary exploratory laparotomy for patients with unresectable tumors, the role of CT in staging gastric cancer has been controversial. The diagnostic accuracy of CT scans in determining the degree of extraserosal invasion and identifying metastatic lymph nodes is still not satisfactory (Sussman, et al. 1988; Fukuya, et al. 1995; Adachi, et al. 1997; Seong, et al. 1988). Recent MR studies regarding the T staging of AGC suggest new possibilities to overcome these limitations of CT (Matsushita, et al. 1994; Oi, et al. 1997; Dux, et al. 1997; Costanzi, et al. 1996). A Japanese group reported high diagnostic accuracy (88% in T staging) from MRI in evaluating extraserosal invasion of AGC using a low signal intensity band on a gradient echo image, which was created by a chemical shift misregistration artifact and a phase cancellation artifact (Matsushita, et al. 1994). In an experimental study, Dux et al. (1997) described that MR staging of gastric cancer was technically possible (accuracy of T staging 65% and of N staging 80%), although they could not reproduce the results of the Japanese group. On the contrary, Costanzi et al. (1996) reported low accuracy of N staging (43%), induced by motion and respiratory artifacts and a long acquisition time. Such discrepancies in diagnostic accuracy of MR staging for gastric cancer are probably due to the variable imaging techniques and criteria of image interpretation.

Post contrast study of stomach show highly enhancement on gastric carcinoma and relatively well delineation of lesion and surrounding fat plain also well demonstrated (Figure 1). In case of serosal involvement of gastric carcinoma, there is fat obliteration of fat plain surrounding tumor (Figure 2).

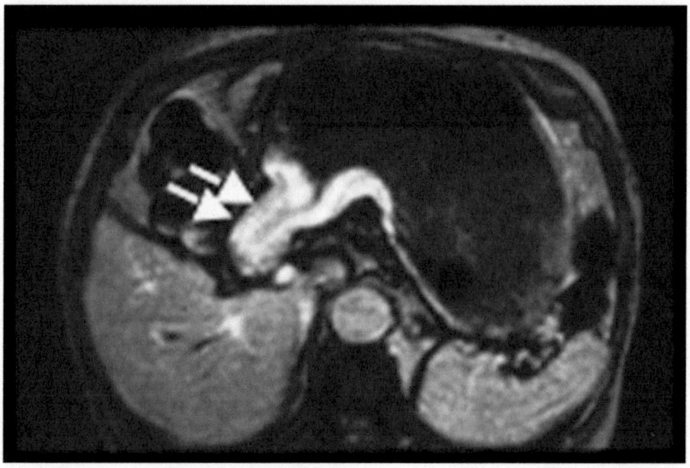

Fig. 1. T2 Gastric Carcinoma. 56-year-old man. Post contrast T1WI image show enhancement of the mass in stomach antrum and relatively preservation of surrounding fat plane (arrows).

Advanced gastric cancer presented as a thickened wall showing varied contrast enhancement from strong to minimal on MR imaging. According to Sohn et al. (2000) study, one of eight cases of early gastric cancer is detected on MR imaging. The tumor detection rate is 73.3% (22/30) on MR imaging. The overall accuracy of MR imaging for the T factor was 73.3% (22/30). On MR imaging, the incidence of under staging was 20% (6/30), whereas

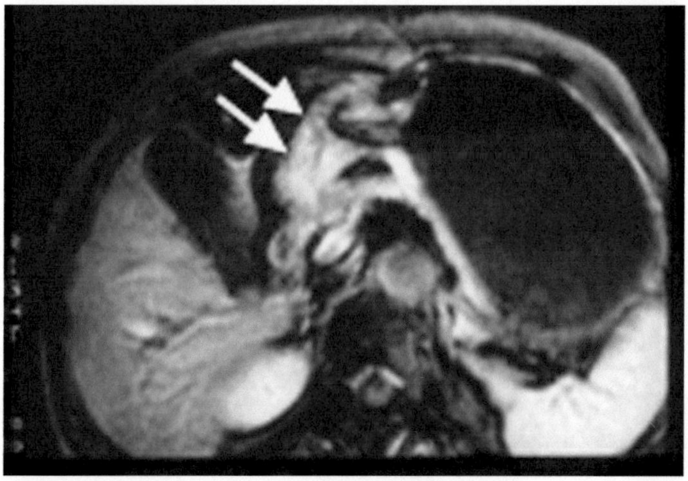

Fig. 2. T3 Gastric Carcinoma. 62-year-old woman. Post contrast T1WI show enhanced mass in stomach antrum and obliteration of pancreatic fat plane, but this case confirmed T3 gastric carcinoma without invasion of pancreas (arrows).

that of over staging was 6.7% (2/30). MR imaging is correct in 60% (18/30) of cases. The MR imaging findings are concordant with the pathologic findings for 87.5% (7/8) of pT1 tumors, 66.7% (2/3) of pT2 tumors, 78.6% (11/14) of pT3 tumors, and 40% (2/5) of pT4 tumors. One pT2 tumor is under staged as MRT1, two pT3 tumors are under staged as MRT2, and three of the pT4 tumors are under staged as MRT3. One pT1 tumor is over staged as MRT2, and one pT3 tumor is over staged as MRT4 (Figure 3). MR can delineate pancreatic invasion (Figure 4).

MR imaging showed the 80% detection rate of omental tumor infiltration. Peritoneal carcinomatosis is poorly delineated on MR imaging. Kim A et al. (2000) reported the study that comparative studies between MR and CT of gastric cancer. In this study, a markedly thickened wall considered as a cancerous lesion on MR images and in total T staging, MRI showed superior results to CT (81 vs. 73%).

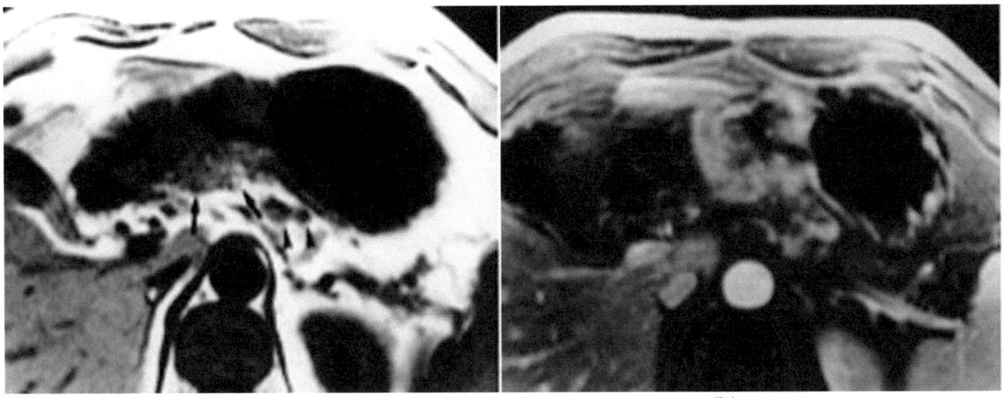

(a) (b)

Fig. 3. T3 Gastric Carcinoma. 54-year-old man. A, B. Axial unenhanced (A) and contrast-enhanced (B) T1-weighted MR images show concentric tumor with strong contrast enhancement in gastric body. Extraluminal nodule of gastric tumor and infiltration in adjacent fat (arrows, A) are well seen on A. Note few enlarged lymph nodes in left perigastric region (arrowheads, A) (Sohn, et al. 2000).

According to Kim A et al. (2000) study, MRI was superior to CT in T staging (overall accuracy 81%; $p < 0.005$). Several cases were overestimated with CT also in the present study, and they were mostly the pT2 cases. Six cases of pT2 were interpreted as T3 or T4 on CT scan due to the streaky densities in perigastric fat surrounding the gastric mass or due to the direct continuity between the gastric mass and the adjacent organs. This finding may have been induced by the partial volume-averaging effect of the angled gastric portion or by the associated perigastric inflammatory change (Sussman, et al. 1988; Minami, et al. 1992). Among these six patients, two were correctly diagnosed by MRI. This fact suggests that MRI can be potentially useful in providing multiplanar images and various pulse sequences compared with CT. Surgical resection clearly is the only potentially curative therapy for gastric cancer. Therefore, under any circumstances, there is no doubt that surgical resection is the best treatment of choice for patients with AGC whenever possible. In practice, accurate T staging can be less meaningful to surgeons when it is below T3 as the method of surgical resection does not change depending on the T stage (Siewert, et al. 1993). The differentiation between T3 and T4 is of more value to surgeons and patients prior to

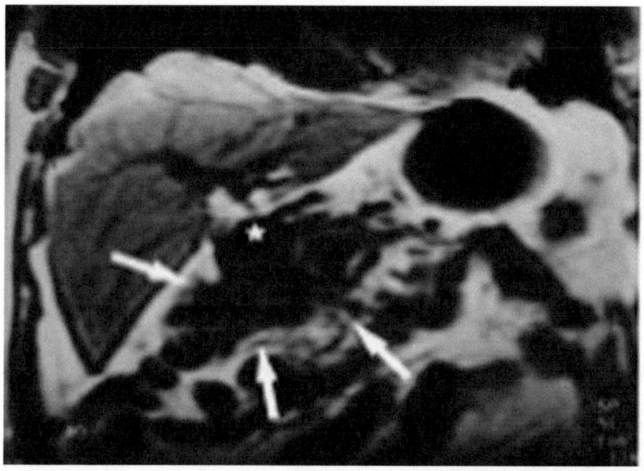

Fig. 4. T4 Gastric Carcinoma. 54-year-old woman. Coronal T1-weighted MR image shows matted appearance of gastric tumor, duodenal loop, and omentum of hepatic flexure of colon (MRT4) (*arrows*). These structures adhered to each other and were infiltrated by tumor, as noted at surgery (pT4). Star indicates pyloric antrum of stomach (Sohn, et al. 2000).

surgery. In Kim, A. et al (2000) study, unfortunately, cases with pathologic T4 were excluded because most patients who were diagnosed as T4 on preoperative imaging studies did not undergo surgery. Although Kim A et al. (2000) could not demonstrate the comparative data between the two imaging modalities in T4 staging, MRI seems to be superior to CT in T4 staging according to previously published data (diagnostic accuracy 75-80 vs. 58-75%) (Oi, et al. 1997; Dux, et al. 1997; Adachi, et al. 1997; Fukuya, et al. 1997; Cho, et al. 1994).

3.2.1 Signal intensity characteristics of normal gastric wall

Interest in the use of MRI for the staging of gastric carcinoma is increasing, but most clinical studies stage the local tumor situation without the differentiation of gastric wall layers (Sohn, et al. 2000; Goldberg & Thoeni. 1989; Halvorsen & Thomson. 1991; Campeau et al. 1995). Studies that use depiction of gastric wall layers as a basis for local tumor staging and lymph node metastasis are rare (Palmowski, et al. 2006; Dux, et al. 1997). The high quality of soft-tissue imaging of MR systems enables the depiction of anatomic wall layers. Auh et al. (1994) studied the gastric wall using an experimental 4.7-T system whereas Lubienski et al. (2002) used an experimental 2.4-T system. Both groups proved that the depiction of gastric-wall layers is technically possible. Auh et al. (1994) depicted 3 layers whereas Lubienski et al. (2002) was able to differentiate 4 layers and correlated them to the mucosa, lamina muscularis mucosa, submucosa and muscularis propria. Typically 3 gastric wall layers are visible. The inner layer corresponds to the mucosa and lamina muscularis mucosa and the middle layer to the submucosa. The outer layer showed the same SI as the muscularis propria in the study of Lubinski's et al. (2002) and therefore mainly consisted of muscle tissue and serosal layers. Palmowski et al. (2006) demonstrated that a reliable depiction of gastric-wall layers can be achieved by a conventional 1-T MRI. As no subserosa and serosa could be depicted, it must be presumed that they were located on the outer side of the third layer. So the third layer represented the muscularis propria, subserosa, and serosa together

(Palmowski, et al. 2006). Dux et al. (1997) proved that under experimental conditions, up to five layers of the gastric wall can be differentiated on MR imaging as they can in endoscopic sonography.

On MRI, two to three layers with different SI in the normal gastric wall can be depicted (Kim, I., et al. 2009). However, there was a mainly three-layered structure (multilayered pattern) of the gastric wall by MRI. The inner layer showed an increase of SI and was 1-3 mm thick on the T1-weighted images. The second had a lower SI with thickness that varied at different sites in the same individual. The outer layer showed a slightly higher SI. On T2-weighted images, the inner and outer layers regularly had a low SI, and the middle layer a high SI. On the basis of the comparison, these three layers were considered to correspond histologically to the mucosal, submucosal, and muscularis propria and serosal layers, respectively (Figure 5).

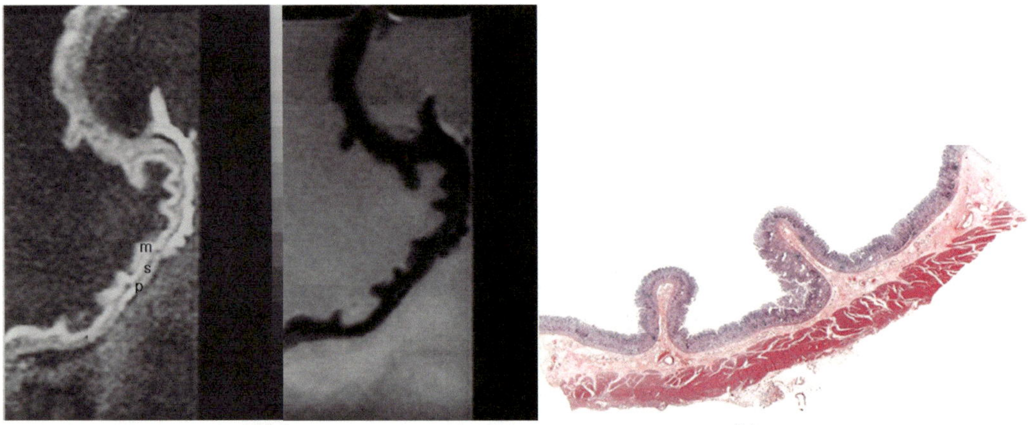

(a) (b)

Fig. 5. MRI and Histology of Normal Gastric Wall. A: T1-weighted (500/20) sagittal image of resected gastric wall showed three layers. The inner layer corresponds to the mucosa (m) and the middle layer to the submucosa(s). The outer layer basically consists of the muscularis propria (p) from which the serosa cannot be differentiated; B: T2-weighted (2500/90) MR image showed low SI on mucosa and muscularis propria and relatively high SI on submucosa; C: Light microscopic section of normal gastric wall obtained from the greater curvature site of stomach body showed three layers which are compatible with inner mucosal layer, middle submucosa layer and outer muscularis propria and serosal layer (H-E stain; original magnification, × 1) (Kim, I., et al. 2009).

Kim I et al. (2009) reported that the inner and outer layers as hyperintense and the middle layer as hypointense at 1.5-MRI. When the three layers were depicted in the gastric wall, the mucosa and the muscularis propria were clearly different from the intervening submucosal layer on T1-weighted images. The distinction among the layers is based mainly on the lower SI of the submucosa compared with that of the mucosa or muscularis propria. The difference between the three layers was also depicted in the T2-weighted images.

3.2.2 Detection of primary tumor

MR imaging of gastric carcinoma on resected specimens studied by Kim I et al. (2009) showed as follows: two cases of Bormann's type 1 carcinoma (polypoid type), seven cases of Bormann's type 2 (ulcerative type), six cases of Bormann's type 3 (ulcerative type with infiltration), and four cases of Bormann's type 4 (infiltrating type). One case of early gastric carcinoma with type IIc was observed, whose lesion was seen as a depression of the mucosa with thinning of the gastric wall on axial and sagittal scanning (Figure 6). Gross pathologic findings showed tumor lesions as follows; two cases of Bormann's type 1, four of Bormann's type 2, nine of Bormann's type 3, four of Bormann's type 4. One case of early gastric carcinoma with type IIc was proved upon histologic examination. The accuracy of MR imaging in the Bormann's type classification was 89% (16 of 19). Differentiation between Bormann's type 2 and type 3 lesions was erroneous in three lesions.

The location of gastric carcinoma was also identified on the MR images. There were nine cases of gastric carcinoma involvement in the gastric antrum, three cases in the stomach body, seven cases in the antrum and the body, one case involving the entire stomach. Upon gross specimen examination, there was no difference between them and the MRIs.

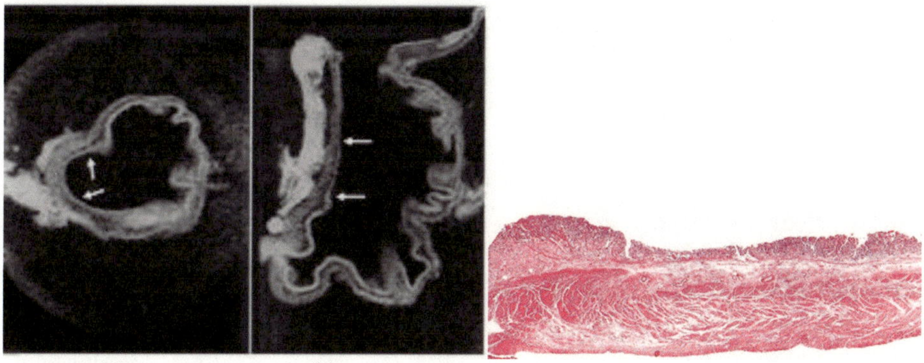

(a) (b) (c)

Fig. 6. MRI and Histology of Early Gastric Carcinoma. A: T1-weighted (500/20) axial image showed depression of gastric wall and obliteration of submucosal low SI (arrows); B: T1-weighted sagittal MR image showed depressed mucosa with tumor invasion to submucosa layer (arrows); C: Light microscopic section showed depressed mucosa with tumor invasion to submucosa (H-E stain; original magnification, × 1) (Kim, I., et al. 2009)).

3.2.3 Depth of tumor invasion

According to Kim I et al. (2009) study, MRIs of gastric carcinoma in resected specimens showed various findings, including thickening of the gastric wall with irregularity in the mucosal SI obliteration, thickening of the gastric wall with first and second layer SI obliteration, diffuse thickening of the gastric wall with third layer SI obliteration and irregularity with ulceration as well.

T1-weighted images showed intermediate SI in regions affected by gastric carcinoma compared to the surrounding normal mucosa and muscularis propria SI. T2-weighted images showed low SI in the gastric carcinoma. Most tumors had a homogenous SI. However, in some cases necrosis and calcification caused an inhomogeneous SI. It is not possible to differentiate between the muscularis propria, subserosa, and serosa. The reason for this inability was that Kim I et al. (2009) considered the subserosa and serosa as being located on the outer border of the joint layer representing the muscularis propria, subserosa, and serosa. If an infiltration was visible, the tumor was classified as T2 as long as it did not reach the outer border. Penetration of the external margin meant at once infiltration of the serosa, and the tumor was staged as a T3 carcinoma, according to the AJCC (2002). The MR imaging findings of gastric wall invasion included 1 case of T1, 7 of T2 (Figure 7), and 11 of T3 (Figure 8). Pathologic results of resected specimens included 3 cases of pT1, 4 of pT2, and 12 of pT3. Differentiation between T1 and T2 classifications was not difficult in cases displaying a distinction between three layers. However, two cases of pT1 were over staged as T2. One case of pT2 was over staged as T3. Two cases of pT3 were under staged as T2. Differentiation between T2 and T3 lesions was difficult due to the outer muscularis propria and serosal layer's thinness and could not always be demonstrated by MRIs. The level of accuracy in determining the T factor according to the TNM classification was 74% (14 of 19 lesions).

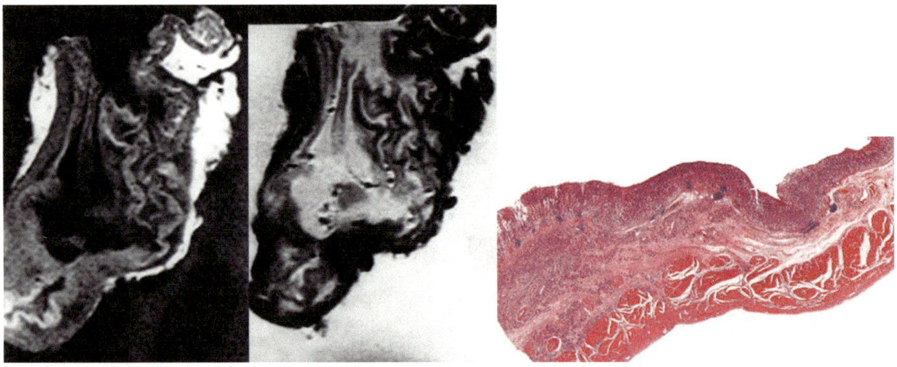

(a) (b) (c)

Fig. 7. MRI and Histology of T2 Gastric Carcinoma. A: T1-weighted (500/20) sagittal image showed diffuse thickening of gastric wall with obliteration of mucosa, submucosa and muscularis propria SI in antrum and lower body, while preserved outer marginal SI; B: T2-weighted (2000/90) sagittal MR images showed ill defined lesion with minimal increased and same SI compared to surrounding normal gastric wall; C: Light microscopic section demonstrate proper muscle invasion of gastric cancer (H-E stain; original magnification, × 1) (Kim, I., et al. 2009).

Palmowski et al. (2006) reported that carcinomas show an intermediate SI on T1-weighted images, a low SI on T2-weighted images and a high SI on opposed phase images. Opposed phase images were not obtained in Kim I et al. (2009) study, but Dux et al. (1997) demonstrated that opposed phase images show a very high SI in gastric tumors and insisted that this was useful for the staging of gastric carcinoma. In Kim I et al. (2009) study, the infiltration of gastric carcinoma was correctly defined in 74% of the cases. This was not different from that of CT images that had an accuracy rate of 50%-85% and that of MR images that had an accuracy rate of 73% (Sohn, et al. 2000; Botet,et al. 1991; Kim, A., et al. 2000). Yamada et al. (2001) reported that gastric specimens that were imaged after fixation in formalin and then MR imaged could also depict early gastric carcinoma.

Kim I et al. (2009) demonstrate that the inner and outer layers as hyperintense and the middle layer as hypointense at 1.5-MRI. When the three layers were depicted in the gastric wall, the mucosa and the muscularis propria were clearly different from the intervening submucosal layer on T1-weighted images. The distinction among the layers is based mainly on the lower SI of the submucosa compared with that of the mucosa or muscularis propria. The difference between the three layers was also depicted in the T2-weighted images. In this

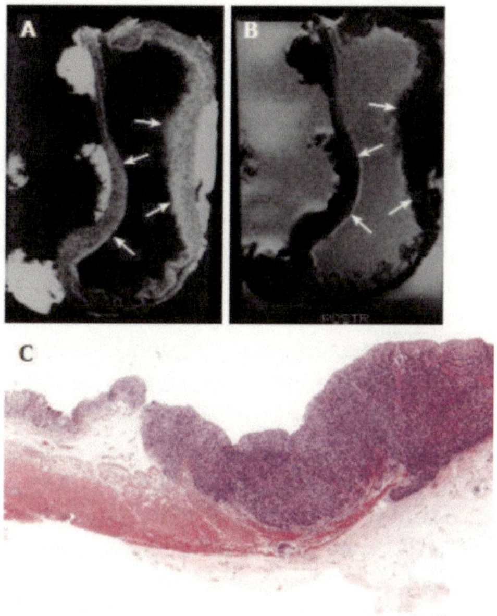

→

Fig. 8. MRI and Histology of T3 Gastric Carcinoma. A: T1-weighted (500/20) sagittal image showed thickening of gastric wall with all three layer SI change in lesser and greater curvature site of stomach body (arrows); B: T2-weighted (2000/90) sagittal MRI showed minimal increase of SI on lesion site and poor delineation of gastric wall SI at out layer margin compared to normal gastric wall (arrows); C: Light microscopic section showed extension of tumor invasion to serosal layer (HE stain; original magnification, × 1) (Kim, I., et al. 2009) .

study, gastric carcinomas appeared as masses with destruction of the normal structure of the gastric wall or diffuse thickening of the gastric wall and showed intermediate SI compared to surrounding normal gastric walls on T1-weighted images and low SI on T2-weighted images. Both sequences were useful for tumor localization and complement each other because some carcinomas in the study could only be recognized by deviating signal behavior in one of the 2 sequences. In Kim I, et al. (2009) study, signal characteristics of the carcinoma depending on the MR sequence were not analyzed. In this study, one case of early gastric carcinoma was depicted on MRI with a shallow depressed wall. This was made possible by adequate distention of the resected stomach with saline.

CT is the most frequently used imaging technique for the staging of gastric cancer. Cho et al. (1994) and Fukuya et al. (1997) studied using dynamic or helical CT and reported that the normal gastric wall frequently showed a two- or three-layer pattern that was interrupted by a tumor; thus, more accurate staging of the T factor could be expected. In addition, the use of thin collimation (≤5 mm) could improve the depiction of small lesions and make it possible to obtain multiplanar reformatted images. However, it still is difficult for helical CT to differentiate between a pT2 tumor and a pT1 tumor with massive submucosal invasion because the hypoattenuating stripe corresponding to the intact submucosal layer could be obliterated in the latter (Fukuya, et al. 1997). Sohn et al. (2000) also experienced a case of a pT2 tumor with minimal invasion of the muscularis propria layer, which showed focal wall thickening with preservation of the hypoattenuating stripe. In this study, advanced gastric cancer was easily detectable on both MR imaging and helical CT; however, the incidence of detectability of early gastric cancer was low on both techniques. MR imaging was slightly more accurate than helical CT in the T staging of gastric cancer, but this difference was not statistically significant ($p > 0.05$). MR imaging and helical CT showed understaging more frequently than overstaging because of the frequent understaging of pT4 tumors. The low concordance rates of pT4 tumors on MR imaging and helical CT were partly caused by the fact that patients with evident CTT4 or MRT4 tumors did not undergo surgery and therefore were not included in this study. Also, invasion into the transverse mesocolon was difficult to detect. Under normal conditions, the transverse mesocolon can be identified on CT scans and MR images as the fatty plane extending from the pancreas to the transverse colon. However, cachexia and a distended stomach frequently efface this fatty plane in patients with advanced gastric cancer, thereby hindering proper evaluation. For pancreatic invasion, the accuracy was the same for both techniques; however, the number of cases of pancreatic invasion ($n = 2$) was too small to analyze in this study. Lee et al. (1994) suggested the superiority of MR imaging over CT because the difference in signal intensity of the stomach and pancreas could make the detection of tumor invasion into the pancreas easier on MR images. However, further study is needed to evaluate the usefulness of MR imaging for this purpose. Early or miliary peritoneal carcinomatosis without ascites was difficult to detect preoperatively, but omental infiltration was easily detected on both MR imaging and helical CT in most (80%) (Sohn, et al. 2000). Generally, MR imaging is a powerful imaging tool with its high soft-tissue contrast, multiplanar imaging capability and ability to provide biochemical and anatomic information, technical versatility for sequence selection and modification, and its lack of ionizing radiation. However, excessive motion artifacts resulting from a combination of long imaging time and physiologic motion such as respiration, peristalsis, and cardiovascular pulsation, have made MR imaging unsuitable for the staging of gastric cancer. The recent development of fast imaging techniques with breath-hold sequences has allowed rapid data acquisition, thereby reducing the problem of motion artifacts. Additionally, the use of phased array coils has increased the signal-to-noise ratio and the spatial resolution in abdominal MR images. Many kinds of oral contrast agents distend the stomach for MR imaging, and these can be divided into positive (producing high signal intensity on T1- and T2-weighted images), negative (producing low signal intensity on T1- and T2-weighted images), and biphasic (producing opposite signal intensities on T1- and T2- weighted images) contrast agents (Halvorsen, et al. 1996).

4. Imaging findings of regional lymph nodes

4.1 Metastasis to regional lymph nodes

Clinically, N staging appears to be a more significant factor than T staging in determining the type of surgery to be performed and in predicting the patient's prognosis (Belcastro, et al. 1990). In AGC, the importance of noting the nodal stage N2 and differentiating it from the N1 stage is well known. This is because N2 nodes are not routinely removed at surgery and, as a result, are the causes of a large number of treatment failures following surgery (Levine & Megibow. 1994). Nevertheless, there has been no consensus until now as to how to measure lymph nodes (short or long axis) or the size that should be considered pathologic (Trenkner, et al. 1994). Wide ranges of sensitivity (48-91%) have been reported for nodal staging with CT (Sussman, et al. 1988; Botet, et al. 1991; Dehn, et al. 1984; Triller, et al. 1986). Fukuya et al. (1995) suggested that diagnosing lymphadenopathy is problematic for nodes of<14 mm in size: 87.2% were negative for metastases. Hence, they used a size criterion of 15

mm for positive metastatic lymph nodes. However, application of the 15 mm criterion can produce high specificity but can induce low sensitivity in N staging.
8 mm at the short axis of lymph node used as the size criterion (Dorfman, et al. 1991), and the N staging accuracy of spiral CT was slightly superior to that of MRI in Kim A et al. (2000) study ($p > 0.05$). The relatively inferior N staging results of MRI to those of CT were related to a low detection rate of small-sized lymph nodes, as reported by Dux et al. (1997). The accuracy of CT in T and N staging of AGC was also variable in several reports (Cho, et al. 1994; Ziegler, et al. 1993; Minami, et al. 1992) and ranged from 73.1 to 83% in T staging and from 51 to 70% in N staging. According to these reports, CT has a tendency to overestimate T stage and underestimate N stage. Understaging occurs because it is difficult to identify fine metastases including peritoneal carcinomatosis, whereas overstaging occurs due to the obliteration of fat plane between the gastric lesion and adjacent organs, which is known to be an unreliable sign suggesting invasion of the adjacent structure. MR imaging correctly revealed regional lymph node involvement in 55% (16/29), understaged 34.5% (10/29), and overstaged 10% (3/29) according by Sohn et al. (2000). There is no significant difference between MR imaging and helical CT in the staging of regional lymph node metastasis. Lymph nodes showed a high SI on opposed phased images (Dux, et al. 1997). MRI had low rate in depicting lymph node metastasis, with an accuracy of 47 %. MRI can reliably depict several anatomical layers of the gastric wall and also MRI of gastric carcinoma could enable accurate diagnosis of location, gross appearance, degree of gastric wall invasion of the tumors and delineation of regional lymph node metastasis. A clear image of the tumor can be achieved. Therefore, an evaluation of the local tumor stage of gastric carcinoma and Sohn et al. (2000) assumed that MR multiplanar imaging would be more accurate in nodal staging than helical CT with only axial images, but with a relative lack of experience and unfamiliarity with MR anatomy in coronal and sagittal images for lymph node detection, he could not prove the superiority of MR imaging over helical CT in nodal staging. Sohn et al. (2000) also considered the detectability of lymph node metastases would be improved by radiologists having more experience with interpretation of coronal and sagittal MR images. The detection rate of lymph node metastasis was low for both techniques. The low detection rate was due to frequent microscopic nodal invasion and the fact that reactive or inflammatory nodal enlargement could not be differentiated from metastatic nodal enlargement on MR imaging or helical CT. An accurate assessment of metastatic lymph nodes was difficult when they were grouped together or attached to a gastric mass. Though an exophytic tumor growth can sometimes mimic a regional lymph node metastasis on axial helical CT, coronal or sagittal MR imaging can easily differentiate them. Perigastric lymph node metastasis based on morphologic criteria is technically possible. Therefore, the additional application of signal intensity as a pathologic lymph node criterion or additional pulse sequences such as Gd-enhanced, breath-hold gradient echo images with fat suppression or breath-hold short T1 inversion recovery (STIR) images could be helpful in improving N staging with MRI.

4.2 Regional lymph node metastasis of resected stomach

According to Kim I et al. (2009) study, the lymph nodes presented with intermediate SI on T1-weighted images, intermediate SI on T2-weighted images. The sizes were measured as being from 0.35 cm to 3.5 cm on MR imaging (Figure 9, 10). The accuracy of N staging by MRI was 47%.

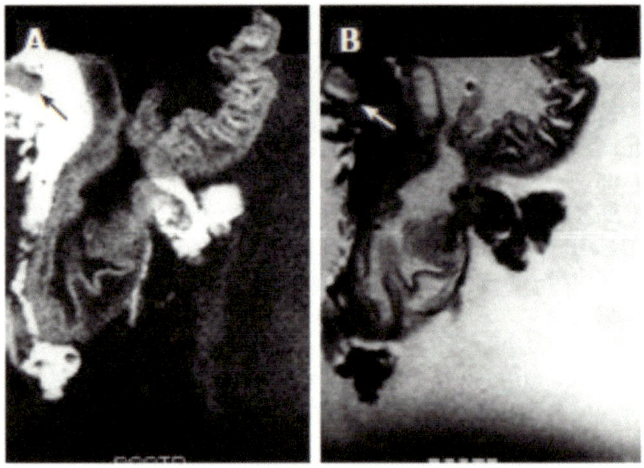

Fig. 9. MRI of N1 Gastric Carcinoma. A: T1-weighted (500/20) MR image showed single lymph node on lesser curvature site of stomach body (Arrow); B: T2-weighted (2000/90) MRI showed intermediated signal SI of lymph node (arrow) (Kim, I., et al. 2009).

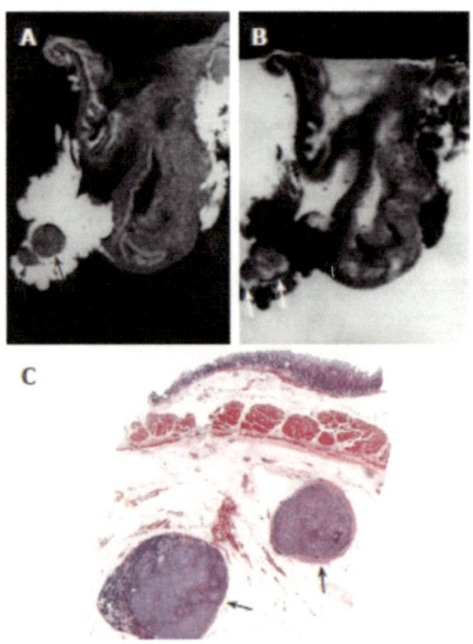

Fig. 10. MRI and Histology of N2 Gastric Carcinoma. A: T1-weighted (500/20) MRI showed two lymph nodes in lesser curvature site of stomach antrum (arrows). Eight lymph nodes are detected in total in perigastric area (not shown); B: T2-weighted (2000/90) MRI showed intermediate SI in the lymph nodes (arrows); C: Light microscopic section showed two lymph nodes in lesser curvature site of gastric antrum (arrows) (HE stain; original magnification, × 1) (Kim, I., et al. 2009).

MRI in combination with standard sequences demonstrated the potential of MRI in the staging of gastric carcinomas. Although the result obtained in N-staging was not acceptable, it should be explored further. However, there could be shown not only MR findings of gastric wall invasion but also perigastric lymph node involvement in the gastric carcinoma. MRI is useful for staging of T staging of gastric cancer, whereas MRI has shown some limitations in N staging. MRI can not completely replace spiral CT in staging AGC at the present time. However, MRI can be potentially useful as an alternative method of staging gastric cancer in that it provides multiplanar images. The evaluation of lymph node metastasis on MRIs had some limitation (Kim, I., et al. 2009), since the size criteria was used only on MRIs and there was no trial of contrast enhancement because of *in vitro* study of gastric carcinoma. Lymph node borders and signal intensity were not also evaluated for diagnosis of lymph node metastasis. But some cases of lymph nodes showed intermediate SI on T1 and T2-weighted images in the tumor infiltration region and this was correctly correlated with the histology. According to Dux et al. (1997) study, lymph nodes showed a high SI on opposed phased images. MRI had low rate in depicting lymph node metastasis, with an accuracy of 47 %. However, the result was similar to the other reports (Yamada, et al. 2001). MRI can reliably depict several anatomical layers of the gastric wall and also MRI of gastric carcinoma could enable accurate diagnosis of location, gross appearance, degree of gastric wall invasion of the tumors and delineation of regional lymph node metastasis. A clear image of the tumor can be achieved.

5. Discussion

Gastric carcinomas show an intermediate SI on T1-weighted images, a low SI on T2-weighted images and a high SI on opposed phase images (Palmowski, et al. 2006). Opposed phase images show a very high SI in gastric tumors and insisted that this was useful for the staging of gastric carcinoma (Dux, et al. 1997) and demonstrate that the infiltration of gastric carcinoma was correctly defined in 74% of the cases. Cho et al. (1994) and Fukuya et al. (1997) studied using dynamic or helical CT and reported that the normal gastric wall frequently showed a two- or three-layer pattern that was interrupted by a tumor; thus, more accurate staging of the T factor could be expected. In addition, the use of thin collimation (≤5 mm) could improve the depiction of small lesions and make it possible to obtain multiplanar reformatted images. However, it still is difficult for helical CT to differentiate between a pT2 tumor and a pT1 tumor with massive submucosal invasion because the hypoattenuating stripe corresponding to the intact submucosal layer could be obliterated in the latter. Sohn et al. (2000) also experienced a case of a pT2 tumor with minimal invasion of the muscularis propria layer, which showed focal wall thickening with preservation of the hypoattenuating stripe. Sohn et al. (2000) demonstrated that advanced gastric carcinoma was easily detectable on both MR imaging and helical CT; however, the incidence of detectability of early gastric cancer was low on both techniques. MR imaging was slightly more accurate than helical CT in the T staging of gastric cancer, but this difference was not statistically significant ($p > 0.05$).

The evaluation of lymph node metastasis on MRIs had some limitation, since the size criteria was used only on MRIs and there was no trial of contrast enhancement because of in vitro study of gastric carcinoma. Lymph node borders and signal intensity were not also evaluated for diagnosis of lymph node metastasis. But some cases of lymph nodes showed intermediate SI on T1 and T2-weighted images in the tumor infiltration region and this was correctly correlated with the histology. MRI can be shown gastric wall invasion but also perigastric lymph node involvement in the gastric carcinoma. Advances in the variation of sequence techniques, as well as application of ultrafast imaging techniques, may be more useful preoperative staging of gastric carcinomas by MRI. MR imaging could be a useful alternative to helical CT because of its high resolution of soft tissue, its multiplanar imaging capability, and its lack of ionizing radiation. In addition, MR imaging could be useful for patients who cannot undergo CT because of renal impairment, pregnancy, or hypersensitivity to CT contrast materials.

6. References

Adachi, Y., Sakino, I., Matusmata, T., & et al (1997). Preoperative assessment of advanced gastric carcinoma using computed tomography. Am J Gastroenterol 1997; 92:872-880. Bibliographic Links.

American Joint Committee on Cancer (2002). Cancer staging handbook. Philadelphia, Pa: Springer-Verlag, 2002.

Auh, Y., Lim, T., Lee, D., Kim, Y., Lee, M., Cho, K., Mun, C., & Lee, I. (1994). In vitro MR imaging of the resected stomach with a 4.7-T superconducting magnet. Radiology 1994; 191: 129-134.

Belcastro, G., Nicolanti, V., Ferri, M., Chiavellati, L., Fratticioli, C., & Schillaci, A. (1990). Prognostic factors in stomach cancer: invasion of gastric serosa and lymph node involvement [Italian]. Minerva Chir 1990; 45:1287-1291.

Botet, J., Lightdale, C., Zauber, A., Gerdes, H., Urmacher, C., Brennan, M.(1991). Preoperative staging of gastric cancer: comparison of endoscopic US and dynamic CT. Radiology 1991; 181:426-432. Bibliographic Links

Campeau, N., Johnson, C., Felmlee, J., Rydberg, J., Butts, R., Ehman, R., & et al (1995). MR imaging of the abdomen with a phased-array multicoil: prospective clinical evaluation. Radiology 1995; 195:769-776. PMID: 7754009.

Cho, J., Kim, J., Rho, S., Lee, H., Jeong, H., & Lee, C. (1994). Preoperative assessment of gastric carcinoma: value of two-phase dynamic CT with mechanical injection of contrast material. AJR 1994; 163:69–75.

Costanzi, A., Di Cesare, E., Guadagni, S., Masciocchi, C., De Bernardinis, G., & Maurizi Enrici, R. (1996). Gastric adenocarcinoma: magnetic resonance versus surgical staging. Radiol Med 1996; 92:726–730.

Dehn, T., Reznek, R., Nockler, I., & White, F. (1984). The pre-operative assessment of advanced gastric cancer by computed tomography. Br J Surg 1984; 71:413-427.

Dorfman, R., Alpern, M., Gross, B., & Sandler, M.A. (1991). Upper abdominal lymph nodes: criteria for normal size determined with CT. Radiology 1991; 180:319-322.

Douglass, H., & Nava, H.R. (1985). Gastric adenocarcinoma-- management of the primary disease. Semin Oncol 1985; 12: 32-45.

Dux, M., Roeren, T., Kuntz, C., Richter G.M., & Kauffmann G. W. (1997). MRI for staging of gastric carcinoma: first results of an experimental prospective study. J Comput Assist Tomogr 1997; 21:66-73.

Fukuya, T., Hiroshi, H., Hayashi, T., & et al (1995). Lymph-node metastases: efficacy of detection with helical CT in patients with gastric cancer. Radiology 1995; 197:705-711. Bibliographic Links.

Fukuya, T., Hiroshi, H., Kaneko, K., & et al (1997). Efficacy of helical CT in T staging of gastric cancer. J Comput Assist Tomogr 1997; 21:73-81. Ovid Full Text Request Permissions.

Goldberg, H.I., & Thoeni, R.F. (1989). MRI of the gastrointestinal tract. Radiol Clin North Am 1989; 27:805–812.

Hahn, P.F., Star,k D.D., & Glastad, K.(1992). Biliary system, pancreas, spleen, and alimentary tract. In: Stark DD, Bradley WG Jr, eds. Magnetic resonance imaging, 2nd ed. St. Louis: Mosby, 1992:1.

Halvorsen, R., & Thompson, W.M. (1991). Primary neoplasm of the hollow organs of the gastrointestinal tract: staging and follow up. Cancer 1991; 67: 1181–1188. PMID: 1991278.

Halvorsen, R., Yee, J., & McCormick, V.D. (1996). Diagnosis and staging of gastric carcinoma. Semin Oncol 1996; 23:325–335.

Kajitani, T. (1981). The general rules for the gastric cancer study in surgery and pathology. Part I. Clinical classification. Jpn J Surg 1981; 11: 127-139.

Kim, A.Y., Han, J.K., Kim, T.K., Park, S.J., & Choi, B.I. (2000). MR imaging of advanced gastric cancer: comparison of various MR pulse sequences using water and gadopentetate dimeglumine as oral contrast agents. Abdom Imag 2000; 25:7–13.

Kim, A.Y., Han, J.K., Seong, C.K., Kim, T.K., & Choi, B.I. (2000). MRI in staging advanced gastric cancer: is it useful compared with spiral CT? J Comput Assist Tomogr 2000; 24: 389-394.

Kim, I., Kim, S.W., Shin, H.C., Lee, M.S., Jeong D.J., Kim. C. J., & Kim, Y. T. (2009). MRI of gastric carcinoma: Results of T and N-sting in an in vitro study. World J Gastroentrol 2009; 15: 3992-3998.

Lee, J.M., Kim, C.Y., Chun, K.A., Kim, H.S, & Shinn, K.S. (1994). MR imaging of gastric carcinoma: comparison with CT. J Korean Radiol Soc 1994; 31:287–294.

Levine, M.S., & Megibow, A.C. (1994). Gastric cancer. In: Gore RM, Levine MS, Laufer I, eds. Textbook of gastrointestinal radiology. Philadelphia: Saunders, 1994: 660-683.

Matsushita, M., Oi, H., Murakami, T., & et al. (1994). Extraserosal invasion in advanced gastric cancer: evaluation with MR imaging. Radiology 1994; 192:87-91. Bibliographic Links.

Minami, M., Kawauchi, N., Itai, Y., Niki, T., & Sasaki, Y. (1992). Gastric tumors: radiologic-pathologic correlation and accuracy of T staging with dynamic CT. Radiology 1992; 185:173-178. Bibliographic Links.

Oi, H., Mutsushita, M., Murakami, T., & Nakamura, H. (1997). Dynamic MR imaging for extraserosal invasion of advanced gastric cancer. Abdom Imag 1997; 22:35-40. Bibliographic Links.

Palmowski, M., Grenacher, L., Kuntz, C., Heye, T., & Dux, M. (2006). Magnetic resonance imaging for local staging of gastric carcinoma: results of an in vitro study. J Comput Assist Tomogr 2006; 30: 896-902.

Seong, C., Kim, A., Kim, T.K., Song, C., Han, J., & Choi, B. (1998). MR imaging of advanced gastric cancer: comparison between T1-weighted FLASH, T2-weighted TSE, and trueFISP [Korean; English abstract]. J Korean Radiol Soc 1998; 39:1149–1156.

Siewert, J., Bottcher, K., Roder, J.D., Busch, R., Hermanek, P., & Meyer, H.J. (1993). Prognostic relevance of systematic lymph node dissection in gastric carcinoma. German Gastric Carcinoma Study Group. Br J Surg 1993; 80:1015-1058.

Sohn, K.M., Lee, J.M., Lee, S.Y., Ahn, B.Y., Park, S.M., & Kim, K.M. (2000). Comparing MR imaging and CT in the staging of gastric carcinoma. AJR Am J Roentgenol 2000; 174: 1551-1557.

Sussman, S.K., Halvorsen, R.A., Illescas, F.F., Cohn R. H., Saeed M, Silverman P. M. & et al (1988). Gastric adenocarcinoma: CT versus surgical staging. Radiology 1988; 167:335-340.

Trenkner, S.W., Halvorsen, R.A., & Thompson, W.M. (1994). Neoplasms of the upper gastrointestinal tract. Radiol Clin North Am 1994; 32:15-24.

Triller, J., Roder, R., Stafford, A., & Schroder, R. (1986). CT in advanced gastric carcinoma: is exploratory laparotomy avoidable? Eur J Radiol 1986; 6:181-186.

Werthmuller, W.C., & Margulis, A.R. (1991). Magnetic resonance imaging of the alimentary tube. Invest Radiol 1991; 26:195–200.

Yamada, I., Saito, N., Takeshita, K., Yoshino, N., Tetsumura, A., Kumagai, J., & Shibuya, H. (2001). Early gastric carcinoma: evaluation with high-spatial-resolution MR imaging in vitro. Radiology 2001; 220: 115-121.

Ziegler, K., Sanft, C., Zimmer, T., & et al (1993). Comparison of computed tomography, endoscopy, and intraoperative assessment in TN staging of gastric carcinoma. Gut 1993; 34:604-610.

3

PET Imaging in Gastric Carcinoma

Kiyohisa Kamimura and Masayuki Nakajo
Kagoshima University Graduate School of Medical and Dental Sciences
Japan

1. Introduction

Gastric carcinoma is the fourth most common carcinoma in the world, with an estimated one million new cases every year, and it is the second most common cause of death from carcinoma (Ferlay et al., 2010). Surgery is the mainstay of treatment of gastric carcinoma. Despite recent advances in surgical treatment, the overall prognosis of patients with gastric carcinoma has not improved significantly because the neoplasm is often diagnosed at an advanced stage of the disease. Local and systemic recurrences are common, even after complete resection of the primary tumour and regional lymph nodes. Multimodality therapy, consisting of surgery with adjuvant or neoadjuvant radiotherapy, chemotherapy or both, has been used recently as a means to improve the survival rate of patients with gastric carcinoma. Current data suggest that this carcinoma is best managed with a tailored therapeutic regimen based on thorough preoperative staging of the tumour and an understanding of established prognostic factors (Stein et al., 2000).

The International Union Against Cancer (Unio Internationalis Contra Cancrum: UICC) TNM Classification of Malignant Tumours, 7th edition (Sobin et al., 2009), provides the latest, internationally agreed-upon standards to describe and categorise cancer stages and progression. Staging of gastric carcinoma was performed according to the UICC TNM staging for the T stage, N stage and M stage. The T stage refers to the depth of the invasion of the primary tumour, the N stage refers to the number of metastatic lymph nodes and the M stage indicates the presence or absence of systemic metastases (Table 1). For the N stage, the UICC TNM staging detailed in the 7th edition (Sobin et al., 2009) is a classification system based on the number of metastatic lymph nodes, a variable that has proved to be an independent prognostic factor in gastric carcinoma. In contrast, the Japanese Classification of Gastric Carcinoma (JCGC), 13th edition, provides lymph node station numbers for anatomically separate sites of regional lymph nodes (Japanese Gastric Cancer Association [JGCA], 1998). This classification is based on the study of lymphatic flow and surgical results. There was a difference in the two classification systems, particularly regarding lymph node metastasis, but near standardization was reached in 2010. For the year 2011, not enough data have been collected based on the new standards. We describe lymph node metastasis based on the JCGC, 13th edition, which classifies lymph node metastasis according to the anatomic sites of metastatic lymph nodes (Table 2).

Current preoperative staging techniques, such as endoscopy, barium studies, computed tomography (CT) and endoscopic ultrasonography (EUS), are of limited accuracy, and invasive procedures often are used for better assessment of the stage of the disease. Positron emission tomography (PET) has been evaluated recently in the staging of gastric carcinoma.

T – Primary tumor

TX: Primary tumour cannot be assessed
T0: No evidence of primary tumour
Tis: Carcinoma in situ: intraepithelial tumour without invasion of the lamina propria, high grade dysplasia
T1: Tumour invades lamina propria, muscularis mucosae, or submucosa
 T1a: Tumour invades lamina propria or muscularis mucosae
 T1b: Tumour invades submucosa
T2: Tumour invades muscularis propria
T3: Tumour invades subserosa
T4: Tumour perforates serosa or invades adjacent structures
 T4a: Tumour perforates serosa
 T4b: Tumour invades adjacent structures

N – Regional Lymph Nodes

NX: Regional lymph nodes cannot be assessed
N0: No regional lymph node metastasis
N1: Metastasis in 1 to 2 regional lymph nodes
N2: Metastasis in 3 to 6 regional lymph nodes
N3: Metastasis in 7 or more regional lymph nodes
 N3a: Metastasis in 7–15 regional lymph nodes
 N3b: Metastasis in 16 or more regional lymph nodes

M – Distant Metastasis

M0: No distant metastasis
M1: Distant metastasis

Stage Grouping

Stage 0:	Tis, N0, M0	Stage IIIA:	T4a, N1, M0
Stage IA:	T1, N0, M0		T3, N2, M0
Stage IB:	T2, N0, M0		T2, N3, M0
	T1, N1, M0	Stage IIIB:	T4b, N0, M0
Stage IIA:	T3, N0, M0		T4b, N1, M0
	T2, N1, M0		T4a, N2, M0
	T1, N2, M0		T3, N3, M0
Stage IIB:	T4a, N0, M0	Stage IIIC:	T4a, N3, M0
	T3, N1, M0		T4b, N2, M0
	T2, N2, M0		T4b, N3, M0
	T1, N3, M0	Stage IV:	Any T, Any N, M1

Table 1. UICC TNM, 7th edition, staging for gastric carcinoma

Extent of lymph node metastasis (N)

N0: No evidence of lymph node metastasis
N1: Metastasis to Group 1 lymph nodes, but no metastasis to Group 2 or 3 lymph nodes
N2: Metastasis to Group 2 lymph nodes, but no metastasis to Group 3 lymph nodes
N3: Metastasis to Group 3 lymph nodes
NX: Unknown

Table 2. JCGC, 13th edition, N staging for gastric carcinoma

The regional lymph nodes are classified into three groups depending upon the location of the primary tumour. This grouping system is based on the results of studies of lymphatic flow at various tumour sites, together with the observed survival rate associated with metastasis at each nodal station.

2. PET imaging

PET instrumentation has been available for over 35 years. Recently it has become clear that PET, using the glucose metabolism tracer ^{18}F-fluoro-2-deoxy-D-glucose (FDG), will have a major role in the management of patients, particularly in oncology. Imaging with FDG-PET is based on the altered glucose uptake of neoplastic cells (Fig. 1). FDG is a radiolabelled glucose analogue that accumulates in cells after cellular uptake, mainly by glucose transporters (GLUTs) located on the cell membrane and intracellular phosphorylation by hexokinases. GLUT-1 is the main cell surface protein facilitating the active uptake of FDG. Neoplastic cells overexpress GLUT-1 on their membranes, resulting in higher uptake. The expression of GLUT-1 itself correlates with tumour aggressiveness and carcinoma-related mortality (Kawamura et al., 2001).

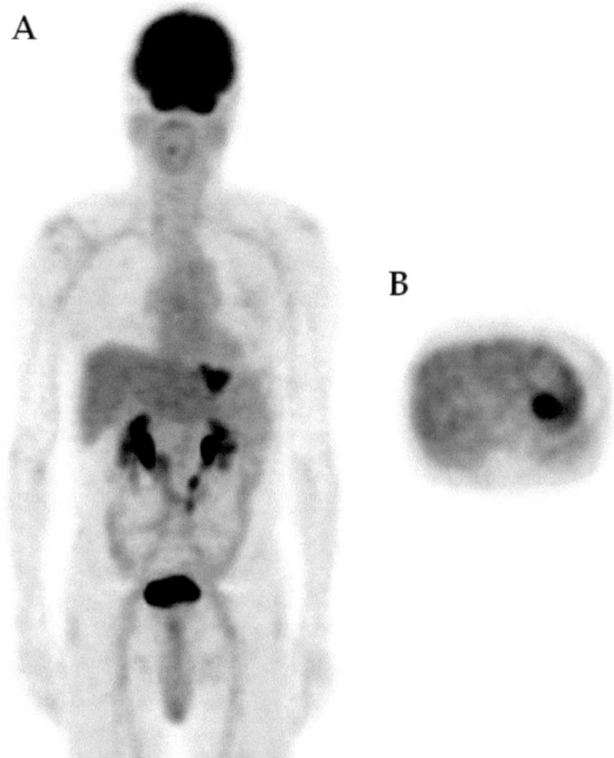

Fig. 1. Representative FDG-PET image of a patient with primary gastric carcinoma. (A) Whole-body anterior projection image of FDG-PET examination highlighting tumour FDG uptake in the gastric wall. (B) Transversal slice of whole-body FDG-PET examination with tumour FDG uptake in the gastric wall.

Apart from visual analysis, an often-used semi-quantitative method to assess the uptake of FDG in a tumour is the standardised uptake value (SUV):

$$SUV = \frac{\text{Regional radioactivity concentration}}{\text{Total injected dose / body weight}}$$ (Lindholmet al., 1993).

This value is the measurement of FDG uptake in a tumour volume normalised on the basis of the distribution volume. SUVs are dependent on several parameters, such as time after FDG injection, tumour size, blood glucose level and spatial resolution of the reconstructed image (Boellaard et al., 2004; Thie, 2004). Relative values, such as SUV changes, measured with accorded and comparable protocols are reliable. Moreover, inter-observer correlations are consistently high (Ott et al., 2003).

2.1 Patient preparation

Patient preparation for a whole-body FDG-PET examination is essential, both to optimise image quality and to minimise physiologic variants and artifacts (Shreve et al., 1999). Patients should fast for a minimum of four hours to ensure that serum glucose and endogenous serum insulin levels are low at the time of FDG administration. Glucose competes with FDG for cellular uptake, and there is some evidence that elevated serum glucose levels will lower the observed FDG uptake in malignant neoplasms (Lindholm et al., 1993). Equally significantly, elevated serum insulin promotes FDG uptake in muscle (Fig. 2. A), so a recent carbohydrate meal or even a snack or the administration of exogenous insulin to lower blood glucose levels can yield extensive muscle uptake. Such muscle uptake will not interfere with the evaluation of centrally located abnormalities such as lung nodules or mediastinal lymph nodes. In general, a serum glucose level of less than 150 mg/dL at the time of FDG accumulation is preferred; a level lower than 200 mg/dL is acceptable. With serum glucose levels above 200 mg/dL, noticeable degradation in image quality due to reduced tissue uptake of FDG and sustained blood pool tracer activity can occur. It is relatively easy to measure serum glucose prior to FDG administration, and this measurement is routine at many centres. Use of exogenous insulin to reduce serum glucose immediately prior to FDG administration is not generally recommended since it will result in accelerated FDG uptake in muscle (Fig. 2. B).

2.2 Image acquisition

2.2.1 Attenuation correction

Whole-body FDG-PET imaging is performed with attenuation correction. As patient movement between the transmission and emission image acquisitions may result in registration artifacts in the attenuation-corrected images, the emission and transmission image acquisitions should be temporally as close as possible when sealed-source transmission scans are used.

2.2.2 Image acquisition time

Image acquisition time and FDG dose are related, but not in the entirely inverse fashion of single-photon radiotracer imaging. Regarding sealed-source transmission scans with image segmentation, acquisition time per bed position is two minutes or less. CT-based attenuation

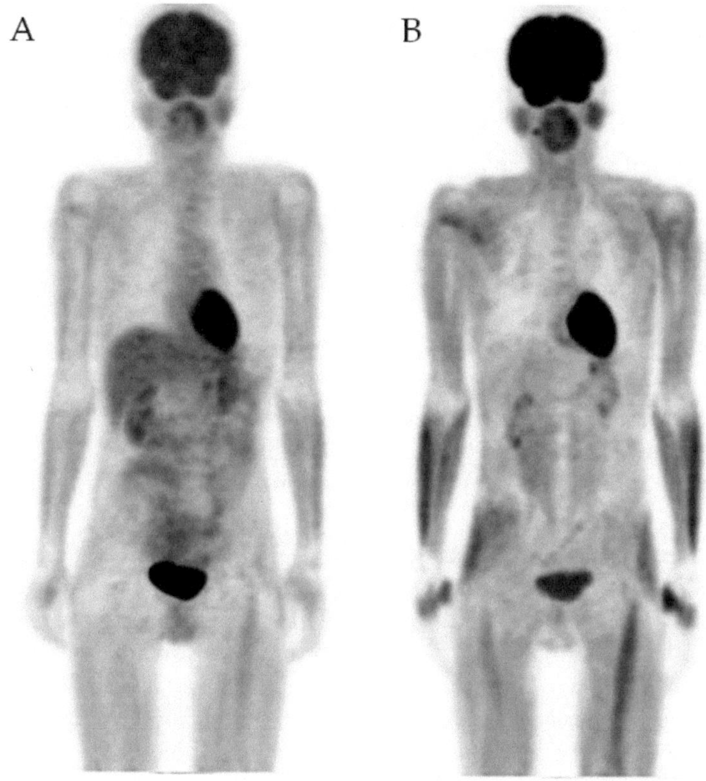

Fig. 2. A and B. Effect of endogenous and exogenous insulin. (A) Whole-body anterior projection image of a patient who ate candies prior to FDG administration and had a serum glucose level of 220 mg/dL, and (B) a patient given 6 units of regular insulin intravenously prior to FDG administration to reach a normalised serum glucose level of 95 mg/dL. In both cases, there is extensive skeletal muscle uptake, uniform and symmetrical, due to the action of insulin.

correction allows a whole-body transmission scan without noise or segmentation errors to be performed in less than 30 seconds with multi-detector helical CT. Shallow relaxed breathing is essential to minimise image registration errors when X-ray CT is used for the transmission image sonogram because when CT acquisition is performed during free breathing, the temporal relation (seconds) is quite different from the PET emission acquisition (a few to several minutes).

2.2.3 Radiopharmaceutical dose

Due to the nature of contaminating scatter and random coincidence events, the relationship between the FDG dose and usable image counting statistics is neither direct nor linear. This relationship depends on the geometry of the tomograph, the type of detector crystal, the size of the patient and the reconstruction algorithm used. In general, ring tomographs in 2D mode with thick axial septa will increase usable true coincidences with increasing administered dose to the upper range of the dosimetry-limited FDG dose (about 700 MBq) (Jones et al., 1982). Increasing the administered dose can reduce the emission image acquisition time, for example, from eight minutes to four minutes per bed position.

Tomographs with greater axial cross-plane acceptance and finer septa, and especially tomographs operating in full 3D mode, will reach limiting random coincidence count rate contributions with administered doses as low as 200 MBq or less.

2.2.4 Time of imaging after tracer injection

Imaging acquisition following FDG administration for body imaging is commenced 40 to 60 minutes following FDG administration. This delay is based in part on the time required for a majority of the activity to clear from the blood pool and for most of the tumour accumulation of the tracer to occur. In fact, there is continued accumulation of FDG in malignant neoplasms and other FDG-avid tissues such as bone marrow beyond one hour, with continued clearance of blood pool activity (Hamberg et al., 1994). Hence, a longer delay in the commencement of image acquisition has been advocated to enhance the tumour-to-background ratio and to allow more complete clearance of upper urinary tract activity. For tomographs that are count-rate limited, a longer delay of 90 to 120 minutes, with a correspondingly higher FDG dose, may provide optimal whole-body imaging.

2.2.5 Imaging display and interpretation

Whole-body FDG-PET images are routinely displayed as a series of orthogonal tomographic images in the transversal, coronal and sagittal planes, together with a whole-body rotating projection image. The rotating projection image provides an invaluable rapid assessment of the overall status of FDG-avid malignancy in the body and can be very helpful in discerning the 3D relationships of abnormalities to normal structures. Interpretation of whole-body images is thus best accomplished using both the rotating whole-body projection image and the serial tomographic images.

Some disagreement remains over the use of semi-quantitative measures of FDG uptake for routine application in oncology, with some centres using SUV routinely and others relying entirely on visual interpretation. SUV cannot be relied upon as an absolute criterion of malignancy because the degree of FGD uptake implies a probability of malignancy rather than an established diagnosis. Even more importantly, the SUVs reported in publications have been obtained using varying methods and do not represent a standardised parameter (Keyes et al., 1995). On the other hand, when a patient undergoes serial PET imaging using the same tomograph in order to assess a change in FDG uptake for therapy monitoring, SUV or a similar semi-quantitative measurement may well be a necessary adjunct to visual interpretation.

2.3 Clinical utility of FDG-PET in gastric carcinoma

2.3.1 Primary tumour staging (T stage)

Most studies included in this review examined the feasibility of primary tumour detection by FDG-PET in gastric carcinoma. The studies show that FDG-PET is not an accurate imaging technique for the primary diagnosis of a gastric primary tumour as it combines high specificity with low sensitivity. About 20% of patients with gastric carcinoma are non-assessable by FDG-PET. The sensitivity rate for detecting the primary tumour varies between 58 and 94% amongst studies (median 81.5%), and the specificity ranges from 78 to 100% (median 98%) (Chen et al., 2005; Mochiki et al., 2004; Mukai et al., 2006; Stahl et al., 2003; Yeung et al., 1998; Yoshioka et al., 2003; Yun et al., 2005). The detection of gastric carcinoma by FDG-PET is complicated by background signalling, partly due to the high physiological uptake of FDG in the normal gastric wall. Moreover, variable and sometimes intense, highly located uptake background activity is observed in the normal gastric wall, resembling false-positive pathological uptake (Mochiki et al., 2004; Stahl et al., 2003). Actively creating gastric distension by water ingestion could augment FDG-PET specificity (Kamimura et al., 2007, 2009; Ott et al., 2003; Yun et al., 2005). After water ingestion, the physiological FDG uptake in the gastric wall became a cystic structure with a mild and even distribution of FDG along the thin wall, and the focal tumour uptake was more clearly visualised under gastric distension by water ingestion (Fig. 3) (Kamimura et al., 2009).

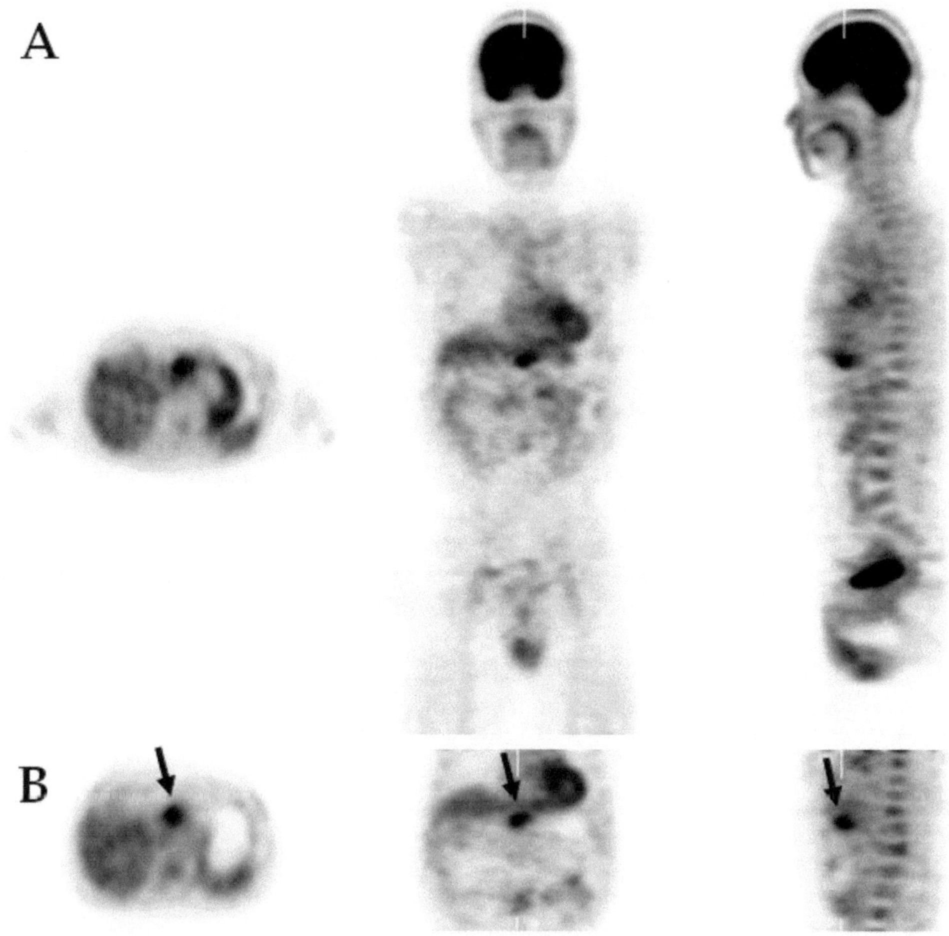

Fig. 3. FDG-PET images of a patient before and after water ingestion. A 63-year-old male with gastric carcinoma of the lower part of the stomach (moderately differentiated tubular adenocarcinoma). Transversal (*left*), coronal (*middle*) and sagittal (*right*) FDG-PET images of the patient. (A) Before ingestion of water, diffuse physiological FDG uptake in the stomach is higher than that in the liver, and it is difficult to distinguish the tumour uptake from physiological FDG uptake in the stomach. (B) After ingestion of water, diffuse physiological FDG uptake in the gastric wall is reduced, and the focal tumour uptake is more clearly visualised (arrows).

Sensitivity of primary tumour identification by FDG-PET is influenced by several other determinants. The location of the tumour (i.e. upper/middle/lower one-third) has been shown to influence the sensitivity of FDG-PET (Mochiki et al., 2004; Mukai et al., 2006; Ott et al., 2003; Stahl et al., 2003). Even in the normal gastric wall, different SUV uptakes have been found between the upper and lower parts of the stomach. Two studies found a higher detection rate by FDG-PET of a gastric carcinoma located in the proximal part of the stomach compared to a distal carcinoma (Koga et al., 2003; Mukai et al., 2006). A second determinant is tumour size or T stage. The sensitivity of FDG-PET ranges from 26 to 63% in early gastric carcinoma (median 43.5%; SUV range 2.1–2.8) to 93–98% in locally advanced gastric carcinoma (median 94%; SUV range 4.3–7.9) (Chen et al., 2005; Mochiki et al., 2004; Mukai et al., 2006; Stahl et al., 2003; Yeung et al., 1998; Yoshioka et al., 2003; Yun et al., 2005). FDG-PET as part of screening programs for the detection of gastric carcinoma in asymptomatic patients yields even worse results (Shoda et al., 2007). A sensitivity of 10% was found, with primarily false-positive findings (Shoda et al., 2007). There are various explanations for this difference. Several studies report a correlation between tumour invasion as an independent factor and overexpression of GLUT-1 receptors. Possibly, the increased need for glucose due to augmented cell metabolism and cell division in advanced carcinoma is the cause of GLUT-1 overexpression and higher FDG uptake (Yamada et al., 2006). The relative volume effect may be a reason for the higher detection rate of advanced gastric carcinoma as the discrimination between physiological and pathological gastric wall uptake increases. This effect makes FDG-PET an inaccurate method for screening and primary tumour detection (Shoda et al., 2007). Furthermore, a clear difference in the sensitivity of FDG-PET is found between different histological carcinoma subtypes. According to the Japanese Classification (JGCA, 1998), gastric carcinoma can be divided into papillary, tubular (well-differentiated type, moderately differentiated type), poorly differentiated (solid type, non-solid type), mucinous adenocarcinoma and signet ring cell carcinoma. The non-intestinal (i.e. diffuse) subtype and carcinomas containing signet ring cells display a consistently low detectability by FDG-PET (Mukai et al., 2006; Ott et al., 2003; Stahl et al., 2003). For tubular adenocarcinoma and moderately differentiated adenocarcinoma, SUV counts of 7.7 to 13.2 were found, which were significantly higher compared to those for mucinous adenocarcinoma and signet ring cell carcinoma (4.1 to 7.7) (Chen et al., 2005; Mochiki et al., 2004; S. K. Kim et al., 2006; Yoshioka et al., 2003; Yun et al., 2005). This result is due to a higher expression of GLUT-1 on the cell membrane of the neoplastic cells, as proven for cohesive gastric carcinoma (i.e. tubular adenocarcinoma, poorly differentiated adenocarcinoma) (Kawamura et al., 2001; W. S. Kim et al., 2000). Other factors influencing the low FDG uptake in mucinous adenocarcinoma and signet ring cell carcinoma are the diffuse growth pattern of non-intestinal gastric carcinoma, the high content of metabolically inert mucus and the low tumour cell density (Kawamura et al., 2001; Ott et al., 2003; Stahl et al., 2003). For these entities, FDG-PET seems to have little value in the primary detection of gastric carcinoma.

2.3.2 Regional lymph node metastases (N stage)

In the N stage, the UICC TNM staging uses a classification system based on the number of metastatic lymph nodes only (Sobin et al., 2009). We describe lymph node metastasis based on the JCGC, 13th edition, which classifies lymph node metastasis according to the anatomic sites of metastatic lymph nodes (JGCA, 1998).

Five studies investigated the value of FDG-PET in detecting lymph node metastasis (Fig. 4) (Chen et al., 2005; S. K. Kim et al., 2006; Mochiki et al., 2004; Mukai et al., 2006; Yun et al., 2005). Sensitivity for metastasis to N1 lymph nodes was very low, ranging from 18 to 46% (median 27.5%) compared to CT (sensitivity of 58–89%; median 68%). This lack of sensitivity could be explained by the relatively low spatial resolution of FDG-PET (5 to 7 mm). The perigastric lymph nodes, therefore, cannot be distinguished from the primary tumour or the normal stomach wall. FDG-PET and CT have low sensitivities of 33–46% and 44–63% in detecting metastases at the N2 and N3 lymph node stations, respectively. Specificity, in contrast, was higher in N1 and N2 lymph node stations with FDG-PET, ranging between 91 and 100% (median 96%), compared to CT (Chen et al., 2005; Mochiki et al., 2004; Mukai et al., 2006; Yun et al., 2005). FDG-PET has a better positive predictive value for lymph node metastasis in comparison to CT, which may alter the planning of therapy, as treatment strategies, especially for N3 lymph node metastasis, change from curative surgery to palliative measures (Chen et al., 2005; Mochiki et al., 2004). A combination of anatomy-based imaging by CT and metabolically based imaging by FDG-PET using PET/CT might, therefore, augment the detection or denial of lymph node involvement.

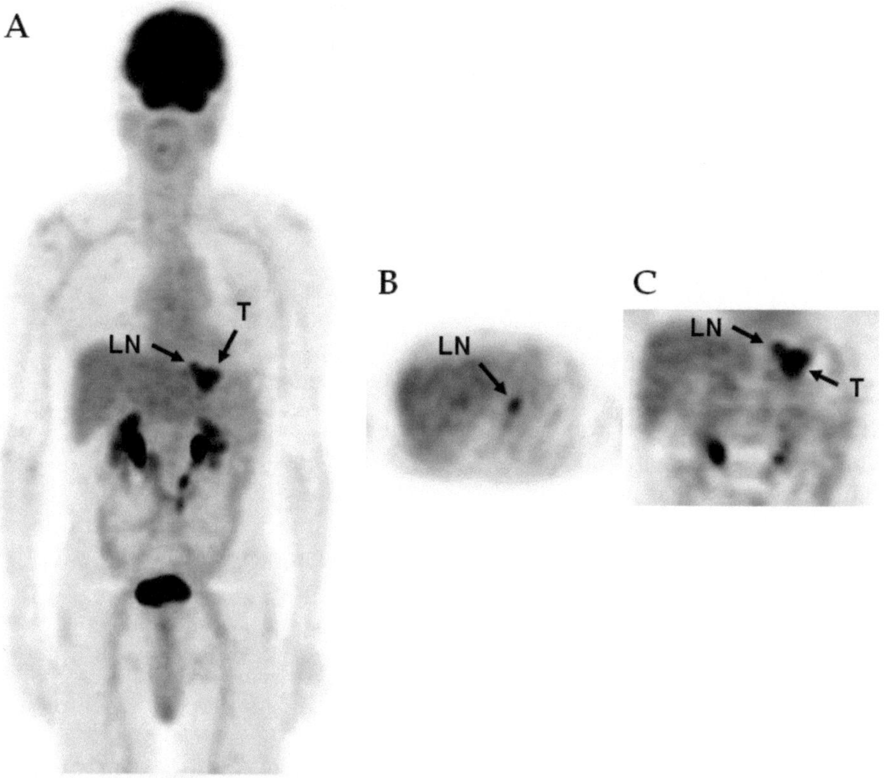

Fig. 4. Representative FDG-PET images of a patient with primary gastric carcinoma with regional lymph node involvement. A 79-year-old male with gastric carcinoma of the upper part of the stomach (moderately differentiated tubular adenocarcinoma). Anterior whole-body projection (A), transversal (B) and coronal (C) FDG-PET images of the patient show intense tumour FDG uptake (T arrows) in the gastric wall and regional lymph node metastasis (LN arrows).

2.3.3 Distant metastatic disease (M stage)

Not much is known about the role of FDG-PET in detecting distant metastasis. However, whole-body FDG-PET can point out distant metastases in some cases (Fig. 5).

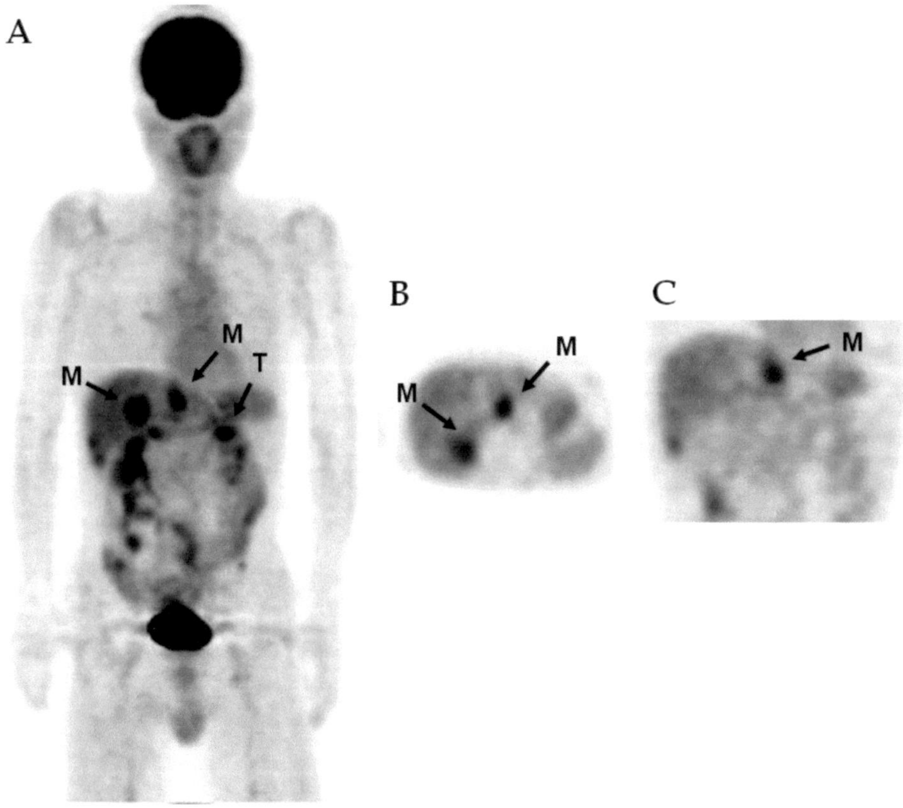

Fig. 5. Representative FDG-PET images of a patient with primary gastric carcinoma with liver metastases. A 75-year-old male with gastric carcinoma of the middle part of the stomach (moderately differentiated tubular adenocarcinoma). Anterior whole-body projection (A), transversal (B) and coronal (C) FDG-PET images of the patient show avid tumour FDG uptake (T arrow) in the gastric wall and multiple liver metastases (M arrows).

One series found respective sensitivities and specificities of 85% and 74% for the detection of liver metastasis, 67% and 88% for lung metastasis, 50% and 63% for peritonitis carcinomatosis, 24% and 76% for ascites, 4% and 100% for pleuritis carcinomatosis and 30% and 82% for bone metastasis (Yoshioka et al., 2003). As is the case for peritoneal carcinomatosis, the low number of metastatic tumour cells in ascites, pleura and bone may explain the low FDG-PET sensitivity. Two patterns of FDG uptake are known to be indicators of peritoneal metastasis: diffuse uptake spreading uniformly throughout the abdomen and pelvis, thus obscuring visceral outlines, and discrete foci of uptake located randomly and anteriorly within the abdomen or independently within the pelvis and unrelated to solid viscera or nodal stations (Lim et al., 2006; Turlakow et al., 2003). Lim et al. demonstrated that although the sensitivity of PET to detect peritoneal metastasis was significantly lower than that of CT (35 vs. 77%), the specificity of PET was significantly higher than that of CT (99 vs. 92%) (Lim et al., 2006). Current CT scanning has poor sensitivity as well, showing specificity even worse than that of FDG-PET. Diagnostic laparoscopy still plays an undefined role in staging gastric carcinoma. It is highly sensitive for peritoneal metastasis detection; however, it has little value in predicting regional lymph node metastasis (Burke et al., 1997; Lowy et al., 1996). The risks and morbidity of a staging laparoscopy outweigh the benefits, as eventually only a small number of patients will benefit from it (Lehnert et al., 2002). With the higher sensitivity of CT and the higher specificity of PET, fusion of these imaging modalities may be more useful than either one alone. In case of suspicion of peritoneal carcinomatosis based on PET and/or CT, diagnostic laparoscopy could be performed to prevent unnecessary laparotomies.

2.3.4 Assessment of response to therapy

The use of neoadjuvant chemotherapy in the treatment of gastric carcinoma has evolved greatly in recent years (Cunningham et al., 2006; Hartgrink et al., 2004; Schuhmacher et al., 2001). Better surgicopathological results could be obtained with this treatment modality, especially by reducing microscopically irradical resections, residual tumour positive lymph nodes and tumour invasion in adjacent organs upon surgery. It is vital to discriminate between responders and non-responders to chemotherapy, as chemotherapy in the latter group could result in unnecessary risk for therapy-related morbidity with co-existing tumour growth. In 80% of all patients, gastric tumours are assessable by FDG-PET, and around 30–40% of gastric carcinoma patients are responders with current chemotherapy regimens as defined by tumour regression (Di Fabio et al., 2007; Ott et al., 2003). Histopathological complete tumour regression is infrequently found (Cunningham et al., 2006; Hartgrink et al., 2004; Ott et al., 2003; Schuhmacher et al., 2001). Thoracoabdominal CT scanning is commonly used to monitor tumour response. CT-observed tumour response depends on tumour size reduction, which is a relative late sign of response (RECIST criteria) (Therasse et al., 2000). An earlier sign of response is chemotherapy-induced reduction in tumour metabolic rate, which can be detected by FDG-PET. Two relatively small studies (44 and 22 patients) showed that the fractional change in glucose consumption could be assessed by FDG-PET immediately following the first cycle of chemotherapy (Di Fabio et al., 2007; Ott et al., 2003). Moreover, FDG-PET has been shown to be a predictor of not only neoadjuvant chemotherapy-induced clinical and histopathological response but also overall survival (Di Fabio et al., 2007; Ott et al., 2003). Patients with a metabolic response had a two-year survival rate of 90%, in contrast to 40% in non-responders (Ott et al., 2003). In addition, 100% of the non-responders were detected by FDG-PET and were subsequently withdrawn from neoadjuvant therapy in order to proceed to immediate surgery. FDG-PET evaluated treatment correctly in ~80% of responders and non-responders combined (Di Fabio et al., 2007; Ott et al., 2003). Future goals are the delineation and validation of SUV-decrement thresholds with adequate sensitivity and specificity to discriminate between beneficiaries and non-beneficiaries of neoadjuvant chemotherapy. Currently, a 35% decrease in SUV as the cut-off level shows 75% sensitivity (Di Fabio et al., 2007; Ott et al., 2003). The role of FDG-PET in monitoring tumour response in gastric carcinoma must be examined further, with the potential for clinically interesting results.

2.3.5 Detection of recurrent disease

Tumour recurrence is directly associated with gastric carcinoma-related mortality, particularly early recurrence (< 1 year disease-free survival) (Shiraishi et al., 2000).

Peritoneal recurrence is especially common (Shiraishi et al., 2000). No curative treatment modalities are left for these patients, and the aim of care is palliation. An exception to this rule is late recurrence (> 5 years disease-free survival), which coincides with sporadic carcinoma mortality (Shiraishi et al., 2000). The extent of lymph node metastasis at primary diagnosis is the most important independent factor determining the timing of tumour recurrence (Shiraishi et al., 2000). Clinical surveillance is the most frequently used follow-up modality, as current endoscopic and radiologic (ultrasonography, barium study and CT) techniques are not sensitive enough for early recurrence detection and no reliable biochemical markers are known to correlate with recurrence (Jadvar et al., 2003; De Potter et al., 2002). Radiological examination, based on anatomical findings, is limited by postoperative non-cancerous changes. The detection of active neoplastic metabolism theoretically increases the advantage of FDG-PET over CT. However, FDG-PET lacks diagnostic accuracy in the early detection of recurrence, with sensitivity and negative predictive values of 70 and 60%, respectively (Jadvar et al., 2003). The high physiological remnant gastric uptake and the low spatial resolution of current hardware prevent the detection of early recurrence by FDG-PET (Jadvar et al., 2003; Yun et al., 2005). Creating gastric distension by water ingestion increases the ability of FDG-PET to discriminate between physiological and pathological gastric uptake and could reduce false-positivity (Kamimura et al., 2009; Yun et al., 2005). On the other hand, the use of PET/CT fusion images could decrease the number of false-positive FDG-PET scans by locating FDG-avid foci on anatomical landmarks.

2.4 Tumour imaging with other tracers

Other potentially useful PET tracers for the evaluation of gastric carcinoma are 3-deoxy-3-^{18}F-fluorothymidine (FLT) and ^{11}C-choline (choline). FLT is a pyrimidine analogue that has proven to be a stable PET tracer that accumulates in proliferating tissue and malignant tumours (Shields et al., 1998). FLT is a substrate for thymidine kinase 1, which is an enzyme involved in the production of thymidine monophosphate. Hermann et al. performed a pilot study assessing the feasibility of FLT-PET compared to FDG-PET in gastric carcinoma (Herrmann et al., 2007). They found a sensitivity of 100% of FLT-PET for primary tumour detection (60% of tumours were signet ring cell carcinoma), compared to a sensitivity of FDG-PET of 69%. Background activity was low. These findings suggest that FLT-PET is a potentially useful imaging modality for the detection and staging of gastric carcinoma, especially for histologic subtypes with low FDG uptake. Kameyama et al. also reported that the sensitivity of FLT-PET was as high as that of FDG-PET for the detection of gastric carcinoma (Kameyama et al., 2009). The cellular uptake of choline presumably reflects its incorporation into phosphatidylcholine, a cell membrane constituent (Hara et al., 1998). The increased uptake of choline in tumour cells is thought to be related to the high rate of tumour cell duplication and cell membrane biosynthesis. In patients with oesophageal carcinoma, Kobori et al. reported that choline-PET was more sensitive than FDG-PET for detecting very small mediastinal lymph node metastases (Kobori et al., 1999). However, FDG-PET was more sensitive than choline-PET in detecting metastases in the upper abdomen due to intense normal uptake of choline in the liver. On the other hand, Pieterman et al. reported that both FDG and choline-PET visualised primary tumours of thoracic carcinoma but that the detection of lymph node metastases was inferior and the detection of brain metastases was superior to those of FDG-PET (Pieterman et al., 2002). Choline-PET does not appear to have been applied to the evaluation of gastric carcinoma.

Further investigations are needed to determine the value of FLT and choline-PET in gastric carcinoma.

3. Conclusion

FDG-PET has a limited role in primary tumour detection due to its low sensitivity, especially in early and non-intestinal gastric carcinoma. However, gastric distention by oral water may decrease physiological gastric uptake of FDG to result in better diagnostic accuracy for advanced gastric carcinoma. FDG-PET has a slightly better positive predictive value for the detection of lymph node metastasis in comparison to CT; furthermore, it has reasonable sensitivity for liver and lung metastases. FDG-PET, therefore, improves preoperative staging in advanced gastric carcinoma. FDG-PET could have a significant role in monitoring tumour response during neoadjuvant chemotherapy because it adequately detects therapy responders at an early stage. Furthermore, FDG-PET is accurate in predicting histopathological response and even long-term prognosis, making it a valuable adjunct to neoadjuvant gastric carcinoma treatment. The results of positron emission tomography in the evaluation and monitoring of gastric carcinoma may improve in the near future. The use of PET/CT fusion imaging has improved diagnostic performance in several carcinoma types (Czernin et al., 2007), and its use in gastric carcinoma is currently under investigation (Hur et al., 2010). The use of other PET tracers, such as FLT and choline, holds promise for the future. Therefore, continued research into PET imaging in gastric carcinoma should be advocated.

4. Acknowledgment

The authors thank the staff members of the PET Centre, Fujimoto-Hayasuzu Hospital, for their assistance. We also thank the staff members of the Department of Radiology, Kagoshima University Graduate School of Medical and Dental Sciences, for their assistance.

5. References

Boellaard, R.; Krak, N.C.; Hoekstra, O.S. & Lammertsma, A.A. (2004). Effects of noise, image resolution, and ROI definition on the accuracy of standard uptake values: a simulation study. *J Nucl Med*, Vol. 45, No. 9, Sep. 2004, pp. 1519–1527, ISSN: 0161-5505.

Burke, E.C.; Karpeh, M.S.; Conlon, K.C. & Brennan, M.F. (1997). Laparoscopy in the management of gastric adenocarcinoma. *Ann Surg*, Vol. 225, No. 3, Mar. 1997, pp. 262–267, ISSN: 0003-4932.

Chen, J.; Cheong, J.H.; Yun, M.J.; Kim, J.; Lim, J.S.; Hyung, W.J. & Noh, S.H. (2005). Improvement in preoperative staging of gastric adenocarcinoma with positron emission tomography. *Cancer*, Vol. 103, No. 11, Jun. 2005, pp. 2383–2390, ISSN: 0008-543X.

Cunningham, D.; Allum, W.H.; Stenning, S.P.; Thompson, J.N.; Van de Velde, C.J.; Nicolson, M.; Scarffe, J.H.; Lofts, F.J.; Falk, S.J.; Iveson, T.J.; Smith, D.B.; Langley, R.E.; Verma, M.; Weeden, S. & Chua, Y.J. MAGIC Trial Participants. (2006). Perioperative chemotherapy versus surgery alone for resectable gastroesophageal cancer. *N Engl J Med*, Vol. 355, No. 1, Jul. 2006, pp. 11–20, ISSN: 0028-4793.

Czernin, J.; Allen-Auerbach, M. & Schelbert, H. (2007). Improvements in cancer staging with PET/CT: Literature-based evidence as of 2006. *J Nucl Med*, Vol. 48, No. 1, Jan. 2007, pp. 78S–88S, ISSN: 0161-5505.

De Potter, T.; Flamen, P.; Van Cutsem, E.; Penninckx, F.; Filez, L.; Bormans, G.; Maes, A. & Mortelmans, L. (2002). Whole-body PET with FDG for the diagnosis of recurrent gastric cancer. *Eur J Nucl Med Mol Imaging*, Vol. 29, No. 4, Apr. 2002, pp. 525–529, ISSN: 1619-7070.

Di Fabio, F.; Pinto, C.; Rojas Llimpe, F.L.; Fanti, S.; Castellucci, P.; Longobardi, C.; Mutri, V.; Funaioli, C.; Sperandi, F.; Giaquinta, S. & Martoni, A.A. (2007). The predictive value of 18F-FDG-PET early evaluation in patients with metastatic gastric adenocarcinoma treated with chemotherapy plus cetuximab. *Gastric Cancer*, Vol. 10, No. 4, Oct. 2007, pp. 221–227, ISSN: 1436-3291.

Ferlay, J.; Shin, H.R.; Bray, F.; Forman, D.; Mathers, C. & Parkin, D.M. (2010). Estimates of worldwide burden of cancer in 2008: GLOBOCAN 2008. *Int J Cancer*, Vol. 127, No. 12, Dec. 2010, pp. 2893–2917, ISSN: 0020-7136.

Hamberg, L.M.; Hunter, G.J.; Alpert, N.M.; Choi, N.C.; Babich, J.W. & Fischman, J. (1994). The dose uptake ratio as an index of glucose metabolism: useful parameter or oversimplification? *J Nucl Med*, Vol. 35, No. 8, Aug. 1994, pp. 1308–1312, ISSN: 0161-5505.

Hara, T.; Kosaka, N. & Kishi, H. (1998). PET imaging of prostate cancer using carbon-11-choline. *J Nucl Med*, Vol. 39, No. 6, pp. 990–995, ISSN: 0161-5505.

Hartgrink, H.H.; van de Velde, C.J.; Putter, H.; Songun, I.; Tesselaar, M.E.; Kranenbarg, E.K.; de Vries, J.E.; Wils, J.A.; van der Bijl, J. & van Krieken, J.H. Cooperating Investigators of The Dutch Gastric Cancer Group. (2004). Neo-adjuvant chemotherapy for operable gastric cancer: long term results of the Dutch randomised FAMTX trial. *Eur J Surg Oncol*, Vol. 30, No. 6, Aug. 2004, pp. 643–649, ISSN: 0748-7983.

Herrmann, K.; Ott, K.; Buck, A.K.; Lordick, F.; Wilhelm, D.; Souvatzoglou, M.; Becker, K.; Schuster, T.; Wester, H.J.; Siewert, J.R.; Schwaiger, M. & Krause, B.J. (2007). Imaging gastric cancer with PET and the radiotracers 18F-FLT and 18F-FDG: a comparative analysis. *J Nucl Med*, Vol. 48, No. 12, Dec. 2007, pp. 1945–1950, ISSN: 0161-5505.

Hur, H.; Kim, S.H.; Kim, W.; Song, K.Y.; Park, C.H. & Jeon, H.M. (2010). The efficacy of preoperative PET/CT for prediction of curability in surgery for locally advanced gastric carcinoma. *World J Surg Oncol*, Vol. 8, No. 86, Oct. 2010, pp. 1–7, ISSN: 1477-7819.

Hur, J.; Park, M.S.; Lee, J.H.; Lim, J.S.; Yu, J.S.; Hong, Y.J. & Kim, K.W. (2006). Diagnostic accuracy of multidetector row computed tomography in T- and N staging of gastric cancer with histopathologic correlation. *J Comput Assist Tomogr*, Vol. 30, No. 3, May-Jun. 2006, pp. 372–377, ISSN: 0363-8715.

Jadvar, H.; Tatlidil, R.; Garcia, A.A. & Conti, P.S. (2003). Evaluation of recurrent gastric malignancy with [F-18]-FDG positron emission tomography. *Clin Radiol*, Vol. 58, No. 3, Mar. 2003, pp. 215–221, ISSN: 0009-9260.

Japanese Gastric Cancer Association. (1998). Japanese Classification of Gastric Carcinoma - 2nd English Edition. *Gastric Cancer*, Vol. 1, No. 1, Dec. 1998, pp. 10–24, ISSN: 1436-3291.

Jones, S.C.; Alavi, A.; Christman, D.; Montanez, I.; Wolf, A.P. & Reivich, M. (1982). The radiation dosimetry of 2 [F-18]fluoro-2-deoxy-D-glucose in man. *J Nucl Med*, Vol. 23, No. 7, Jul. 1982, pp. 613-617, ISSN: 0161-5505.

Kameyama, R.; Yamamoto, Y.; Izuishi, K.; Takebayashi, R.; Hagiike, M.; Murota, M.; Kaji, M.; Haba, R. & Nishiyama, Y. (2009). Detection of gastric cancer using 18F-FLT PET: comparison with 18F-FDG PET. *Eur J Nucl Med Mol Imaging*, Vol. 36, No. 3, Mar. 2009, pp. 382–388, ISSN: 1619-7070.

Kamimura, K.; Fujita, S.; Nishii, R.; Wakamatsu, H.; Nagamachi, S.; Yano, T.; Ogita, M.; Umemura, Y.; Fujimoto, T. & Nakajo, M. (2007). An analysis of the physiological FDG uptake in the stomach with the water gastric distention method. *Eur J Nucl Med Mol Imaging*, Vol. 34, No. 11, pp. 1815–1818, ISSN: 1619-7070.

Kamimura, K.; Nagamachi, S.; Wakamatsu, H.; Fujita, S.; Nishii, R.; Umemura, Y.; Ogita, M.; Komada, N.; Sakurai, T.; Inoue, T.; Fujimoto, T. & Nakajo, M. (2009). Role of gastric distention with additional water in differentiating locally advanced gastric carcinomas from physiological uptake in the stomach on 18F-fluoro-2-deoxy-D-glucose PET. *Nucl Med Commun*, Vol. 30, No. 6, Jun. 2009, pp. 431–439, ISSN: 0143-3636.

Kawamura, T.; Kusakabe, T.; Sugino, T.; Watanabe, K.; Fukuda, T.; Nashimoto, A.; Honma, K. & Suzuki T. (2001). Expression of glucose transporter-1 in human gastric carcinoma: association with tumor aggressiveness, metastasis, and patient survival. *Cancer*, Vol. 92, No. 3, Aug. 2001, pp. 634–641, ISSN: 0008-543X.

Keyes, J.W. Jr. (1995). SUV: standard uptake or silly useless value? *J Nucl Med*, Vol. 36, No. 10, Oct. 1995, pp. 1836–1839, ISSN: 0161-5505.

Kim, H.J.; Kim, A.Y.; Oh, S.T.; Kim, J.S.; Kim, K.W.; Kim, P.N.; Lee, M.G. & Ha, H.K. (2005). Gastric cancer staging at multi-detector row CT gastrography: comparison of transverse and volumetric CT scanning. *Radiology*, Vol. 236, No. 3, Sep. 2005, pp. 879–885, ISSN: 0033-8419.

Kim, S.K.; Kang, K.W.; Lee, J.S.; Kim, H.K.; Chang, H.J.; Choi, J.Y.; Lee, J.H.; Ryu, K.W.; Kim, Y.W. & Bae, J.M. (2006). Assessment of lymph node metastases using 18F-FDG PET in patients with advanced gastric cancer. *Eur J Nucl Med Mol Imaging*, Vol. 33, No. 2, Feb. 2006, pp. 148–155, ISSN: 1619-7070.

Kim, W.S.; Kim, Y.Y.; Jang, S.J.; Kimm, K. & Jung, M.H. (2000). Glucose transporter 1 (GLUT1) expression is associated with intestinal type of gastric carcinoma. *J Korean Med Sci*, Vol. 15, No. 4, Aug. 2000, pp. 420–424, ISSN: 1011-8934.

Kobori, O.; Kirihara, Y.; Kosaka, N. & Hara, T. (1999). Positron emission tomography of esophageal carcinoma using (11)C-choline and (18)F-fluorodeoxyglucose: a novel method of preoperative lymph node staging. *Cancer*, Vol. 86, No. 9, pp. 1638–1648, ISSN: 0008-543X.

Koga, H.; Sasaki, M.; Kuwabara, Y.; Hiraka, K.; Nakagawa, M.; Abe, K.; Kaneko, K.; Hayashi, K. & Honda, H. (2003). An analysis of the physiological FDG uptake pattern in the stomach. *Ann Nucl Med*, Vol. 17, No. 8, Dec. 2003, pp. 733–738, ISSN: 0914-7187.

Lehnert, T.; Rudek, B.; Kienle, P.; Buhl, K. & Herfarth, C. (2002). Impact of diagnostic laparoscopy on the management of gastric cancer: prospective study of 120 consecutive patients with primary gastric adenocarcinoma. *Br J Surg*, Vol. 89, No. 4, Apr. 2002, pp. 471–475, ISSN: 0007-1323.

Lim, J.S.; Kim, M.J.; Yun, M.J.; Oh, Y.T.; Kim, J.H.; Hwang, H.S.; Park, M.S.; Cha, S.W.; Lee, J.D.; Noh, S.H.; Yoo, H.S. & Kim, K.W. (2006). Comparison of CT and 18F-FDG pet for detecting peritoneal metastasis on the preoperative evaluation for gastric carcinoma. *Korean J Radiol*, Vol. 7, No. 4, Oct.–Dec. 2006, pp. 249–256, ISSN: 1229-6929.

Lindholm, P.; Minn, H.; Leskinen-Kallio, S.; Bergman, J.; Ruotsalainen, U. & Joensuu, H. (1993). Influence of the blood glucose concentration on FDG uptake in cancer--a PET study. *J Nucl Med*, Vol. 34, No. 1, Jan. 1993, pp. 1–6, ISSN: 0161-5505.

Lowy, A.M.; Mansfield, P.F.; Leach, S.D. & Ajani, J. (1996). Laparoscopic staging for gastric cancer. *Surgery*, Vol. 119, No. 6, Jun. 1996, pp. 611–614, ISSN: 0039-6060.

Mukai, K.; Ishida, Y.; Okajima, K.; Isozaki, H.; Morimoto, T. & Nishiyama, S. (2006). Usefulness of preoperative FDG-PET for detection of gastric cancer. *Gastric Cancer*, Vol. 9, No. 3, Sep. 2006, pp. 192–196, ISSN: 1436-3291.

Mochiki, E.; Kuwano, H.; Katoh, H.; Asao, T.; Oriuchi, N. & Endo, K. (2004). Evaluation of 18F-2-deoxy-2-fluoro-D-glucose positron emission tomography for gastric cancer. *World J Surg*, Vol. 28, No. 3, Mar. 2004, pp. 247–253, ISSN: 0364-2313.

Ott, K.; Fink, U.; Becker, K.; Stahl, A.; Dittler, H.J.; Busch, R.; Stein, H.; Lordick, F.; Link, T.; Schwaiger, M.; Siewert, J.R. & Weber, W.A. (2003). Prediction of response to preoperative chemotherapy in gastric carcinoma by metabolic imaging: results of a prospective trial. *J Clin Oncol*, Vol. 21, No. 24, Dec. 2003, pp. 4604–4610, ISSN: 0732-183X.

Pieterman, R.M.; Que, T.H.; Elsinga, P.H.; Pruim, J.; van Putten, J.W.G.; Willemsen, A.T.M.; Vaalburg, W. & Groen, H.J.M. (2002). Comparison of (11)C-choline and (18)F-FDG PET in primary diagnosis and staging of patients with thoracic cancer. *J Nucl Med*, Vol. 43, No. 2, Feb. 2002, pp. 167–172, ISSN: 0161-5505.

Schuhmacher, C.P.; Fink, U.; Becker, B.K.; Busch, R.; Dittler, H.J.; Mueller, J. & Siewert, J.R. (2001). Neoadjuvant therapy for patients with locally advanced gastric carcinoma with etoposide, doxorubicin, and cisplatinum. Closing results after 5 years of follow-up. *Cancer*, Vol. 91, No. 5, Mar. 2001, pp. 918–927, ISSN: 0008-543X.

Shields, A.F.; Grierson, J.R.; Dohmen, B.M.; Machulla, H.J.; Stayanoff, J.C.; Lawhorn-Crews, J.M.; Obradovich, J.E.; Muzik, O. & Mangner, T.J. (1998). Imaging proliferation in vivo with [F-18]FLT and positron emission tomography. *Nat Med*, Vol. 4, No. 11, Nov. 1998, pp. 1334–1336, ISSN: 1061-4036.

Shiraishi, N.; Inomata, M.; Osawa, N.; Yasuda, K.; Adachi, Y. & Kitano, S. (2000). Early and late recurrence after gastrectomy for gastric carcinoma. Univariate and multivariate analyses. *Cancer*, Vol. 89, No. 2, Jul. 2000, pp. 255–261, ISSN: 0008-543X.

Shoda, H.; Kakugawa, Y.; Saito, D.; Kozu, T.; Terauchi, T.; Daisaki, H.; Hamashima, C.; Muramatsu, Y.; Moriyama, N. & Saito, H. (2007). Evaluation of 18F-2-deoxy-2-fluoro-glucose positron emission tomography for gastric cancer screening in asymptomatic individuals undergoing endoscopy. *Br J Cancer*, Vol. 97, No. 11, Dec. 2007, pp. 1493–1498, ISSN: 0007-0920.

Shreve, P.D.; Anzai, Y. & Wahl, R.L. (1999). Pitfalls in oncologic diagnosis with FDG PET imaging: physiologic and benign variants. *Radiographics*, Vol. 19, No. 1, Jan. 1999, pp. 61–77, ISSN: 0271-5333.

Sobin, L.H.; Gospodarowicz, M.K. & Wittekind, C. (2009). *TNM Classification of Malignant Tumours (UICC International Union Against Cancer)* (7th edition). Wiley-Blackwell, ISBN: 978-1-4443-3241-4, New York.

Stahl, A.; Ott, K.; Weber, W.A.; Becker, K.; Link, T.; Siewert, J.R.; Schwaiger, M. & Fink, U. (2003). FDG PET imaging of locally advanced gastric carcinomas: correlation with endoscopic and histopathological findings. *Eur J Nucl Med Mol Imaging,* Vol. 30, No. 2, Feb. 2003, pp. 288–295, ISSN: 1619-7070.

Stein, H.J.; Sendler, A.; Fink, U. & Siewert, J.R. (2000). Multidisciplinary approach to esophageal and gastric cancer. *Surg Clin North Am*, Vol. 80, No. 2, Feb. 2000, pp. 659–686, ISSN: 0039-6109.

Therasse, P.; Arbuck, S.G.; Eisenhauer, E.A.; Wanders, J.; Kaplan, R.S.; Rubinstein, L.; Verweij, J.; Van Glabbeke, M.; van Oosterom, A.T.; Christian, M.C. & Gwyther, S.G. (2000). New guidelines to evaluate the response to treatment in solid tumors. European Organization for Research and Treatment of Cancer, National Cancer Institute of the United States, National Cancer Institute of Canada. *J Natl Cancer Inst*, Vol. 92, No. 3, Feb. 2000, pp. 205–216, ISSN: 0027-8874.

Thie, J.A. (2004). Understanding the standardized uptake value, its methods, and implications for usage. *J Nucl Med*, Vol. 45, No. 9, Sep. 2004, pp. 1431–1434, ISSN: 0161-5505.

Turlakow, A.; Yeung, H.W.; Salmon, A.S.; Macapinlac, H.A. & Larson, S.M. (2003). Peritoneal carcinomatosis: role of (18)F-FDG PET. *J Nucl Med*, Vol. 44, No. 9, Sep. 2003, pp. 1407–1412, ISSN: 0161-5505.

Yamada, A.; Oguchi, K.; Fukushima, M.; Imai, Y. & Kadoya, M. (2006). Evaluation of 2-deoxy-2-[18F]fluoro-D-glucose positron emission tomography in gastric carcinoma: relation to histological subtypes, depth of tumor invasion, and glucose transporter-1 expression. *Ann Nucl Med*, Vol. 20, No. 9, Nov. 2006, pp. 597–604, ISSN: 0914-7187.

Yeung, H.W.; Macapinlac, H.; Karpeh, M.; Finn, R.D. & Larson, S.M. (1998). Accuracy of FDG-PET in gastric cancer. Preliminary experience. *Clin Positron Imaging*, Vol. 1, No. 4, Sep. 1998, pp. 213–221, ISSN: 1095-0397.

Yoshioka, T.; Yamaguchi, K.; Kubota, K.; Saginoya, T.; Yamazaki, T.; Ido, T.; Yamaura, G.; Takahashi, H.; Fukuda, H. & Kanamaru, R. (2003). Evaluation of 18F-FDG PET in patients with advanced, metastatic, or recurrent gastric cancer. *J Nucl Med*, Vol. 44, No. 5, May 2003, pp. 690–699, ISSN: 0161-5505.

Yun, M.; Choi, H.S.; Yoo, E.; Bong, J.K.; Ryu, Y.H. & Lee, J.D. (2005). The role of gastric distention in differentiating recurrent tumor from physiologic uptake in the remnant stomach on 18F-FDG PET. *J Nucl Med*, Vol. 46, No. 6, Jun. 2005, pp. 953–957, ISSN: 0161-5505.

Yun, M.; Lim, J.S.; Noh, S.H.; Hyung, W.J.; Cheong, J.H.; Bong, J.K.; Cho, A. & Lee, J.D. (2005). Lymph node staging of gastric cancer using (18)F-FDG PET: a comparison study with CT. *J Nucl Med*, Vol. 46, No. 10, Oct. 2005, pp. 1582–1588, ISSN: 0161-5505.

4

Novel Biomedical Imaging Approach for Detection of Sentinel Nodes in an Orthotopic Xenograft Rat Model of Human Gastric Carcinoma

Akihito Tsubota, Tomoki Koyama, Yoshihisa Namiki, Norio Tada and Hiroshi Takahashi
Jikei University School of Medicine
Japan

1. Introduction

With advances in endoscopic techniques and the widespread use, detection rates for early gastric carcinoma are increasing, and minimally invasive surgery becomes more important in the treatment. Minimally invasive surgery with less extensive dissection involves avoidance of unnecessary lymphadenectomy, leading to the reduction of postoperative morbidity and mortality rates and the improvement of postoperative quality of life without impairing recurrence-free survival. Sentinel node (SN) biopsy is useful to dissect lymph node (LN) rationally and to avoid unnecessarily extensive lymphadenectomy in surgery for gastric carcinoma, as has been established in breast cancer and melanoma (Krag et al., 1998; Morton, 1992; van der Veen et al., 1994; Veronesi et al., 1997). Thus, SN biopsy could be a promising method for the management of gastric carcinoma. The concept is based on the notion that SNs are the first lymph nodes to which cancer cells metastasize from the primary lesion (Sobin, 2003). The presence of tumor cells in SNs indicates that cancer cells may metastasize to downstream nodes. Conversely, the absence of metastatic tumor cells in SNs indicates that metastasis is unlikely in other nodes. However, a convenient and sensitive method useful for the detection of SNs of gastric carcinoma has not been standardized.

Development of a convenient and sensitive method useful for the detection of SNs will enable surgeons to rationally determine the extent of LN dissection and to perform minimally invasive surgery (Krag et al., 1998; Morton, 1992; van der Veen et al., 1994; Veronesi et al., 1997). Several methods have been developed to detect SNs using radioactive materials or vital dyes, such as patent blue violet, isosulfan blue and indocyanine green in gastric carcinoma (Hayashi et al., 2003; Hiratsuka et al., 2001; Hundley et al., 2002; Ichikura et al., 2002; Isozaki et al., 2004; Karube et al., 2004; Kim, M.C. et al., 2004; Kitagawa & Kitajima, 2002; Lee et al., 2005; Miwa et al., 2003; Nimura et al., 2004; Osaka et al., 2004; Ryu et al., 2003; Simsa et al., 2003; Song et al., 2004; Tanaka et al., 2004). Although the sensitivity of these materials or dyes for the detection of SNs is high, sentinel node navigation surgery using dye- or radio-guided methods has not yet been widely performed in early gastric cancer, partly owing to false-negative results in detecting SNs with tumor cell metastases, or due to their own inherent drawbacks, such as blurred visualization and/or legal restrictions (Hayashi et al., 2003; Hiratsuka et al., 2001; Ichikura et al., 2002; Kim, M.C. et al., 2004; Kitagawa & Kitajima, 2002; Miwa et al., 2003; Tanaka et al., 2004). Accordingly, standardized tracers remain to be determined.

Photosensitizers are used for the treatment of various carcinomas in a remedy that is well known as photodynamic therapy (Fisher et al., 1995; Kvam et al., 1990; Sharman et al., 1999). Photosensitizing agents preferentially accumulate in tumor tissues, and elicit cytocidal effects on tumor cells when excited at a wavelength specific for each agent (Sharman et al., 1999). Photodynamic therapy makes use of photosensitizers with these unique properties to achieve highly selective and localized treatment of various carcinomas (Sharman et al., 1999). ATX-S10Na (II) is a hydrophilic chlorine derivative with a major absorption wavelength of approximately 670 nm, and emits red fluorescence when excited at its absorption wavelength. ATX-S10Na (II) has been developed as a second-generation photosensitizer, which is eliminated more rapidly from the body than previously known first-generation photosensitizers. Therefore, major adverse reactions such as skin photosensitivity have been markedly reduced, compared to those of the first generation photosensitizers (Matsumoto et al., 2003; Mori et al., 2000a, 2000b; Nakajima et al., 1992, 1998). In addition, ATX-S10Na (II) has a high affinity and specificity for tumor tissues, and thereby selectively accumulates in tumor tissues (Matsumoto et al., 2003; Mori et al., 2000a, 2000b; Nakajima et al., 1992, 1998). To our knowledge, our study was the first report that describes the use of a hydrophilic photosensitizer, ATX-S10Na (II), for the detection of SNs in orthotopic transplants of human gastric carcinoma (Koyama et al., 2007a).

In the present chapter, we showed a novel fluorescence-guided imaging system to detect SNs using a photosensitizing agent, ATX-S10Na (II), as a novel fluorescent tracer, and its usefulness for a fluorescence-guided lymphatic mapping system in an animal model of human gastric carcinoma. In the model, human gastric carcinoma cells were implanted orthotopically into nude rats. ATX-S10Na (II) was injected subserosally into the primary tumor lesion, and visualized by a fluorescence spectrolaparoscope. ATX-S10Na (II) would serve as a novel tracer in sentinel node navigation surgery for gastric carcinoma.

1.1 Concept of sentinel node

The sentinel node (SN) is defined as the first lymph node (LN) to receive lymphatic drainage from a primary tumor, and therefore it is commonly accepted that SN is the first LN in which tumor cells from the primary lesion form lymphatic metastases (Sobin, 2003; Fig. 1). Detection of a metastatic tumor in the SN could mean metastasis of tumor cells to the downstream LNs. Conversely, absence of metastatic tumors in the SN indicates that the downstream LNs most likely do not contain metastatic tumor cells.

2. Photosensitive fluorescent tracer

ATX-S10Na (II) [13,17-bis(1-carboxypropionyl) carbamoylethyl-8-ethenyl-2-hydroxy-3-hydroxy-iminoethylidene-2,7,12,18-tetramethyl-prophyrin tetrasodium salt], is synthesized, purified and supplied by Photochemical Co. (Okayama, Japan). Its structure ($C42H41N7Na4$ $O12$; molecular weight 927.77, Fig.2) and metabolism were described in detail previously (Matsumoto et al., 2003; Mori et al., 2000a, 2000b; Nakajima et al., 1992, 1998). When the photosensitizer is activated by irradiation with excitation light of 450±40 nm (mean ± SD), it emits a strong red fluorescence of 667 nm wavelength (Fig. 3). Therefore, we are able to

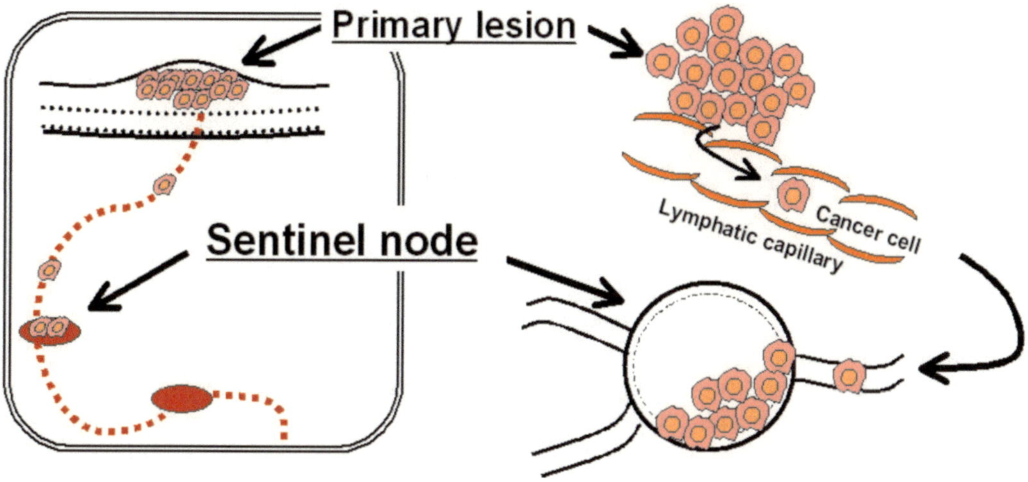

Fig. 1. Concept of sentinel node

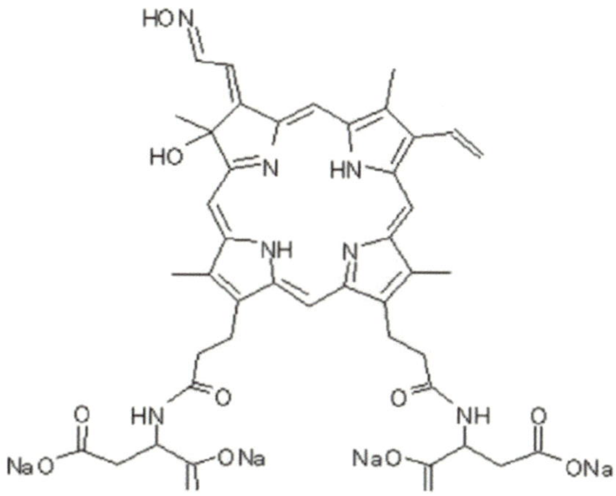

Fig. 2. Chemical structure of ATX-S10Na(II)

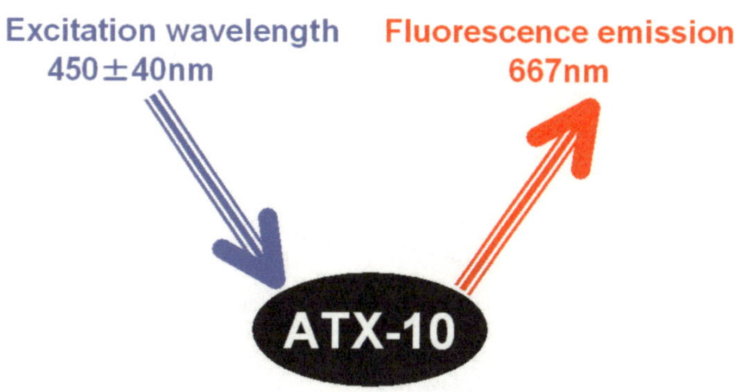

Fig. 3. Basic principle of photosensitizer

detect the sentinel node by the red fluorescence of ATX-S10Na (II) which is injected at the primary tumor. The reagent is stored as a powder in the dark at -80°C, and dissolved in phosphate-buffered saline to a final concentration of 5 mg/ml each time immediately before use.

3. Orthotopic xenograft model of human gastric carcinoma

3.1 Cell line

The OCUM-2M LN cell line was originally derived from human scirrhous gastric carcinoma (Fujihara et al., 1998). This cell line forms LN metastases, when it is injected orthotopically into the stomach of athymic nude rats. Cells are cultured in Dulbecco's modified Eagle's medium (DMEM) supplemented with 10% fetal calf serum, 100 U/ml penicillin, and 100 mg/ml streptomycin in a humidified atmosphere containing 5% CO_2 at 37°C. The cells in the log phase of growth are washed twice with phosphate-buffered saline, treated with trypsin and collected by centrifugation. The cell pellets are dissolved in DMEM and adjusted at a concentration of 5×10^7 cells/ml. Cells are used in the experiments only when their viability exceeds 95%, as determined by the trypan blue dye-exclusion test.

3.2 Tumor cell implantation

Five- to seven-week-old female athymic nude rats (F344/N Jcl-*rnu*; CLEA Japan, Co., Tokyo, Japan) are housed in a temperature-controlled pathogen-free facility, maintained on a 12-hour light/12-hour dark cycle, and provided with commercially available rat chow and tap water *ad libitum*. Rats are pretreated by irradiation with 3 Gy of X-rays 3 days before tumor cell inoculation to reduce the number of active natural killer lymphocytes (Fig. 4). Rats are anesthetized for all procedures by an intraperitoneal injection of pentobarbital sodium (40 mg/kg body weight), and then an incision is made in the upper abdominal median line. The stomach is exposed, and a total of 1×10^6 OCUM-2M LN cells in a volume of 20 µl of DMEM is injected subserosally into the middle anterior wall of the lesser curvature of the stomach with a 29-gauge needle. After the orthotopic implantation of tumor cells, the abdominal wall is sutured and closed using 6-0 surgical sutures. All procedures are performed in a pathogen-free environment. To monitor the growth of inoculated tumor cells, sera are obtained by periorbital bleeding weekly, and the serum levels of CA19-9, a marker of tumor growth, are

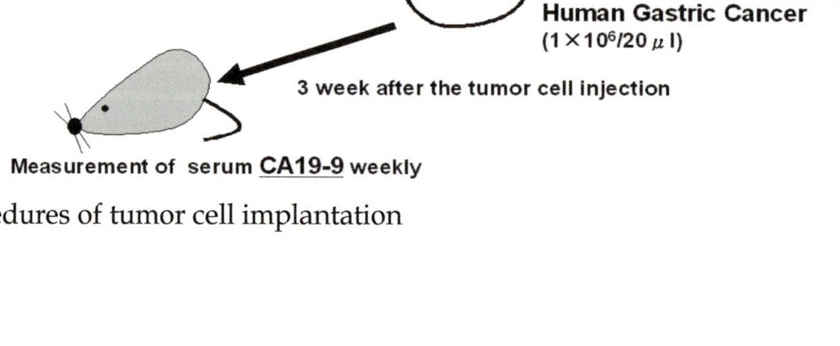

Fig. 4. Procedures of tumor cell implantation

measured by radioimmunoassay using a commercially available kit (Fujirebio, Inc., Tokyo). When the level of serum CA19-9 values increases above 6 units/ml, which is a sign of tumor growth, the presence of SNs is investigated with a fluorescence spectrolaparoscope.

3.3 Establishment of orthotopic xenograft

In our experiment, 95% of nude rats inoculated with tumor cells showed the establishment of orthotopic xenografts of human gastric carcinoma (Koyama et al, 2007a). The primary lesions of the implanted tumors grew up to the median size of 5.0 mm (range, 2.2–8.2 mm) by the largest diameter. In tumor-bearing rats, the median size of the left gastric LNs (Lg-LNs) was 3.9 mm (range, 2.5-14.3 mm) in diameter. Fig. 5 shows a representative example of the primary lesion in the stomach and the enlarged Lg-LN. Subserosally inoculated OCUM-2M LN cells developed into a solid tumor ("primary lesion"; Fig. 5, black arrowhead) at the middle anterior wall of the lesser curvature of the stomach. Enlarged Lg-LN (Fig. 5, white arrowhead), which had tumor metastases, was also observed. The corresponding Lg-LN specimen displays poorly differentiated adenocarcinoma, which is a characteristic feature of OCUM-2M LN, human scirrhous carcinoma of the stomach (Fig. 6; bar = 100 μm).
To confirm the presence of tumor cells in LNs (LN metastasis), human β-actin was amplified specifically by cDNA synthesis of total RNA extracted from tissue samples and subsequent reverse transcriptase-polymerase chain reaction (RT-PCR). The LN metastases were histopathologically observed in 56% of tumor-bearing rats. These tissues were positive for human β-actin by RT-PCR (Koyama et al, 2007a). Control rats did not develop solid tumors and showed no changes in the lymphatic system.

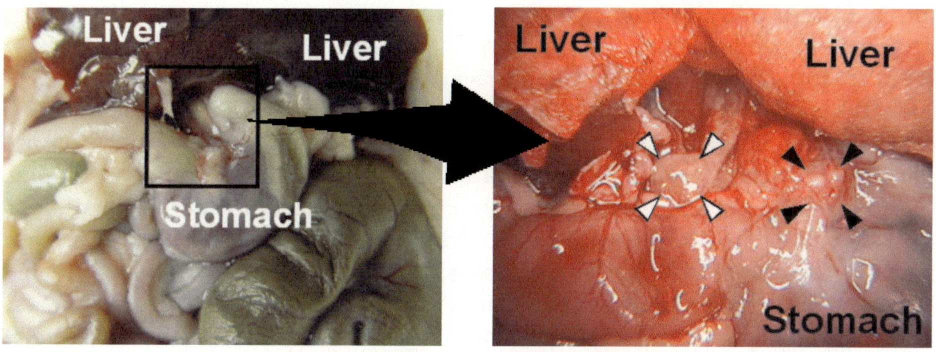

Fig. 5. Establishment of orthotopic xenograft model of human gastric carcinoma

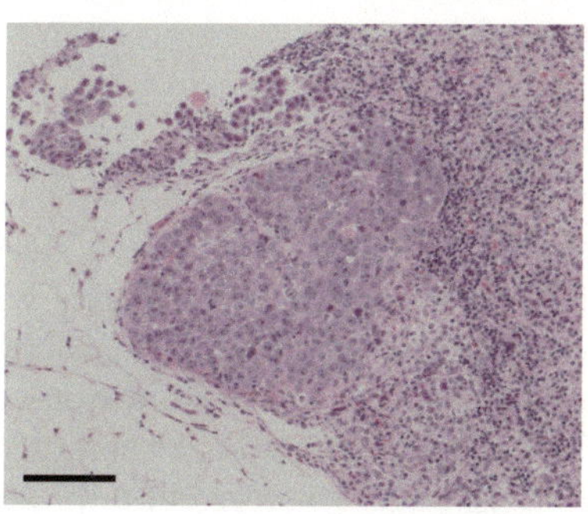

Fig. 6. Hematoxylin and eosin stain of left gastric lymph node

4. Detection of sentinel nodes by fluorescence spectrolaparoscope

4.1 Fluorescence spectrolaparoscope

Re-laparotomy is performed on tumor-implanted rats under general anesthesia, when serum CA19-9 concentrations increase above 6 units/ml. After an exposure of the stomach, ATX-S10Na(II) solution at a total volume of 40–60 μl is injected using a 29-gauge needle into the serosal side of the implanted tumor [Fig. 7(a)]. ATXS10Na(II) injected into the primary lesion is excited by the light of 450±40 nm [Fig. 7(b), 7(c) and 7(d)], which is emitted from the tip of the laparoscope equipped with a xenon lamp and a bandpass excitation filter of 450±40 nm. ATX-S10Na (II) localized in tissues emits fluorescence of 667 nm, which is visualized using a bandpass emission filter of >510-nm. The emission filter is useful for blocking the excitation light and other components such as natural autofluorescence of the surrounding tissues. An image-intensified charge-coupled device (CCD) camera is furnished with two built-in filters, a conventional white-light filter and an emission filter of >510-nm, and is attached to the ocular end of the laparoscope through the adaptor. The dynamic image of excited ATX-S10Na(II) is monitored in real-time on an RGB display via an image processing system, and recorded on a camcorder with 192×10^4 pixels for 60 minutes after the injection. The intensity and exposure time of the excitation light are constant throughout these experiments.

4.2 Dynamic imaging and distribution of photosensitizer

Fluorescence distribution of ATX-S10Na(II) in the abdomen is visualized as vivid red color on the imaging board using the spectrolaparoscope. In tumor-bearing rats, ATX-S10Na (II) solution is injected into the tumor of primary lesion via stomach serosa using a 29-gauge syringe [Fig. 7 (a); white arrowhead]. The red-fluorescent ATX-S10Na(II) is clearly identified and uptaken rapidly into the lymphatic tissue around the primary lesion [Fig. 7 (b)]. Subsequently, the red-emitting fluorescence is incorporated rapidly into the Lg-LN [Fig. 7 (c) and (d); white arrowhead] through the afferent lymphatic vessels [Fig. 7 (c) and (d); white arrows]. The migration of ATX-S10Na(II) takes place within a period of 5 minutes of the injection. The fluorescence intensity increases, reaching a peak and plateau approximately at 1–9 minutes, and persists without attenuation during the entire observation time. In contrast, no or little fluorescence is detected in the surrounding non-lymphatic tissues. The contrast between the red fluorescent tissues and non-fluorescent area is distinct, and all investigators can identify the red fluorescent nodes easily. In control rats, fluorescent dye is incorporated rapidly into the lymph vessels around the injection site, migrates through them and disappears within 3 minutes. Of note, none of the LN is stained with the fluorescence in the control rats.

4.3 Sentinel nodes and nodal metastases

According to the sentinel node (SN) concept, the first LN into which ATX-S10Na(II) flows is regarded as the "SN". Fig. 8 shows an example in which ATX-S10Na (II) was incorporated rapidly into afferent lymphatic vessels around the primary lesion, lymphatic network, and flowed first into the Lg-LN. Thus, the Lg-LN was regarded as the SN. The Lg-LN was occupied with tumor cell metastases, showing poorly differentiated adenocarcinoma with a characteristic feature of OCUM-2M LN, human scirrhous carcinoma of the stomach [Fig. 8 (d); hematoxylin and eosin stain], and was visualized by the red-fluorescence of ATX-S10Na (II) [Fig. 8 (a), (b) and (c)]. The incision was made in the isolated red-fluorescent Lg-LN at

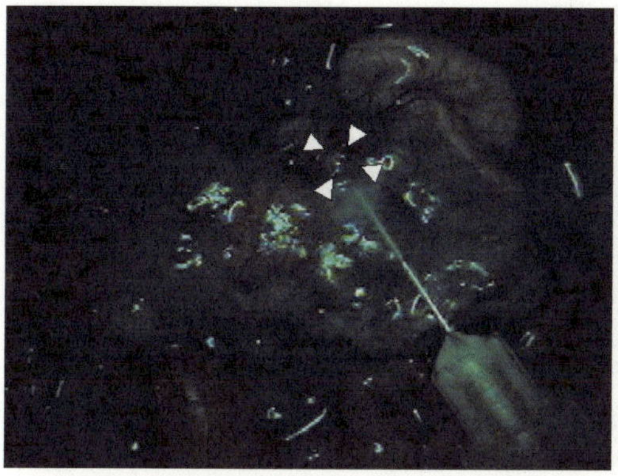

(a) Injection of ATX-S10Na(II)

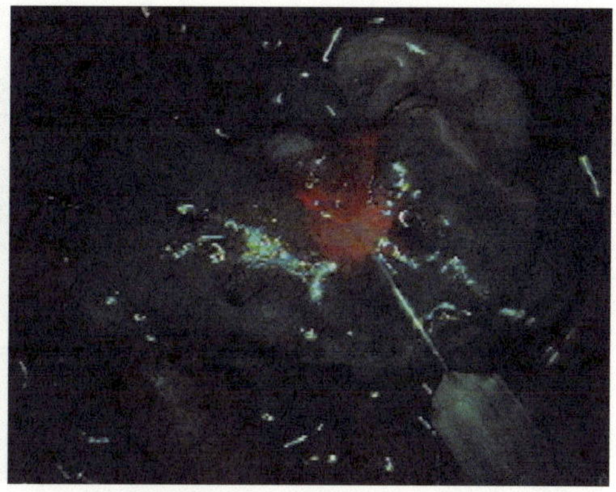

(b) Uptake into lymphatic tissue

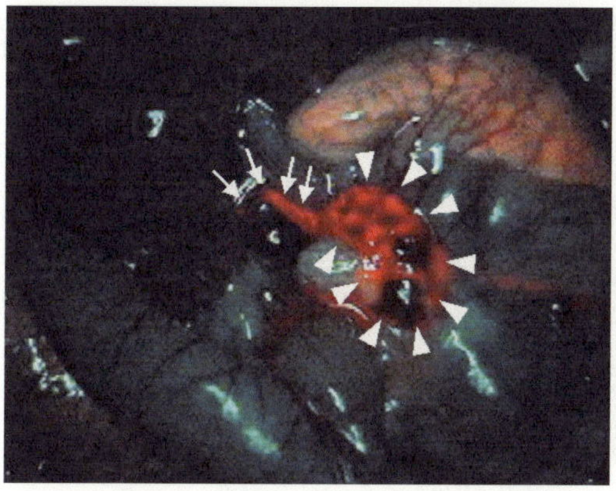

(c) Visualization of lymph nodes

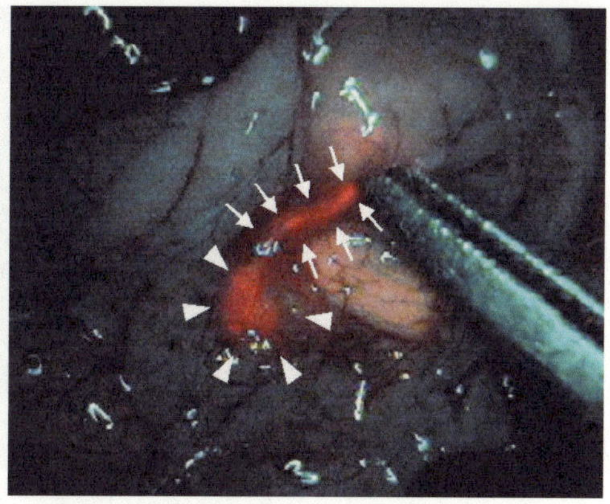

(d) Visualization of lymph nodes

Fig. 7. Detection of lymphatic tissues by ATX-S10Na(II)

the dotted line [Fig. 8 (b)], and the uptake of red fluorescence into metastatic lesion was observed as shown in Fig. 8 (c) and (d). We provisionally termed the red-fluorescent LNs "red nodes", similar to those designated as "blue or green nodes" using vital dyes (Hayashi et al., 2003; Hiratsuka et al., 2001; Ichikura et al., 2002) or "hot nodes" using radioactive particles (Hayashi et al., 2003).

After the completion of each experiment, the Lg-LN (SN) was separated, and the other LNs located downstream of Lg-LN or SN, including the hepatic, splenic and pancreatico-duodenal LNs, were harvested *en bloc*. In all LN samples dissected, the presence of human β-actin mRNA was investigated by RT-PCR to assess the presence of metastases of tumor cells (Koyama et al., 2007a). In 25 out of 27 rats, ATX-S10Na (II) was incorporated into the Lg-LN (SN), which was identified as a red node. Of note, human β-actin was positive in 24 out of these 25 red nodes (SNs). To our surprise, human β-actin was also positive in all LNs located downstream of human-β-actin-positive red-fluorescent Lg-LNs (SNs) in these 24 rats. In contrast, human β-actin was negative in the downstream LNs of the rat with a human-β-actin-negative red-fluorescent Lg-LN (SN). In the remaining 2 out of 27 rats, the ATX-S10Na (II) was incorporated into the hepatic LNs (SNs), but not into the Lg-LN (non-SN). Therefore, the hepatic LN but not the Lg-LN was identified as a red node (SN) in these two rats. Interestingly, both of the two non-red Lg-LNs (non-SNs) were negative for human

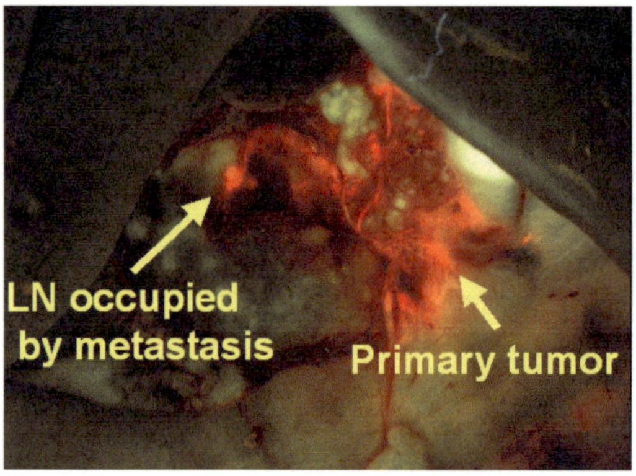

(a) Uptake of ATX-S10Na(II)

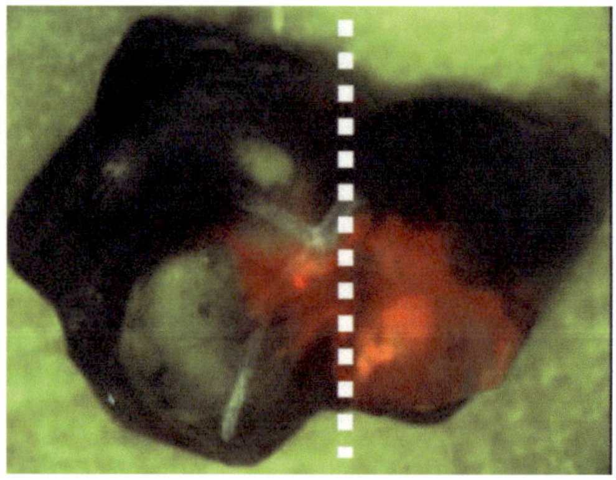

(b) Incision into isolated Lg-LN

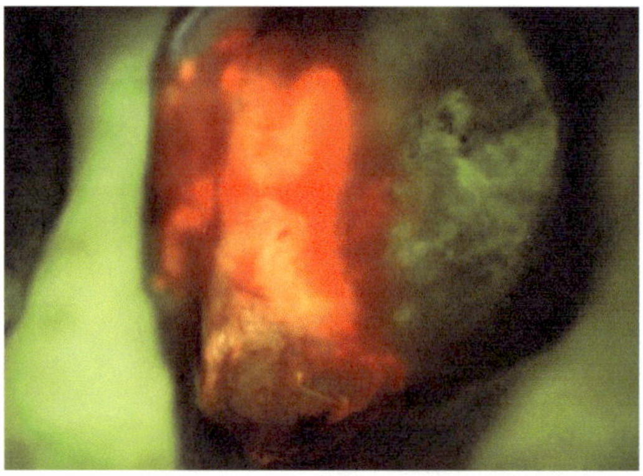

(c) Incised side of isolated Lg-LN

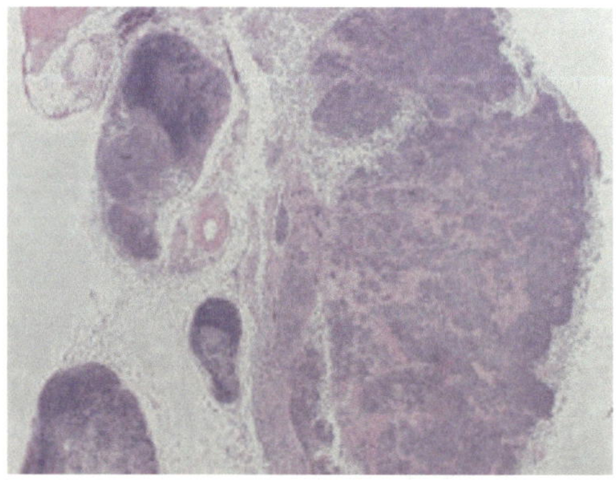

(d) Histopathological findings

Fig. 8. Lymph nodes detected by ATX-S10Na(II)

β-actin, whereas both of the two red-fluorescent hepatic LNs (SNs) were positive for human b-actin. On the single-section specimens, 19 human-β-actin-positive red-fluorescent Lg-LNs were poorly differentiated adenocarcinoma, and others showed no malignant findings. In control rats, human β-actin was negative in both Lg-LNs and other LNs.

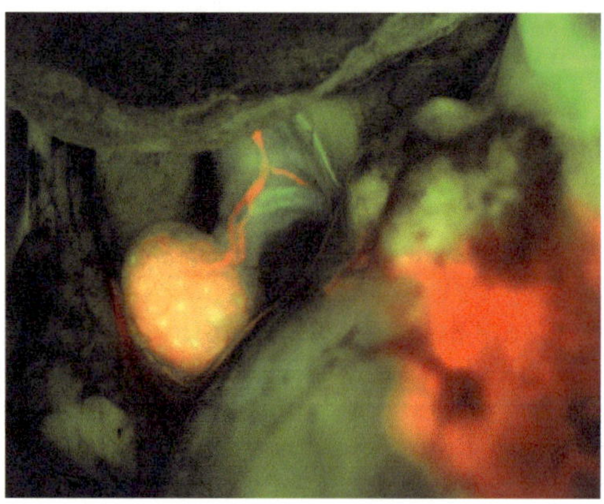

Fig. 9. Uptake of ATX-S10Na(II) in Case 1

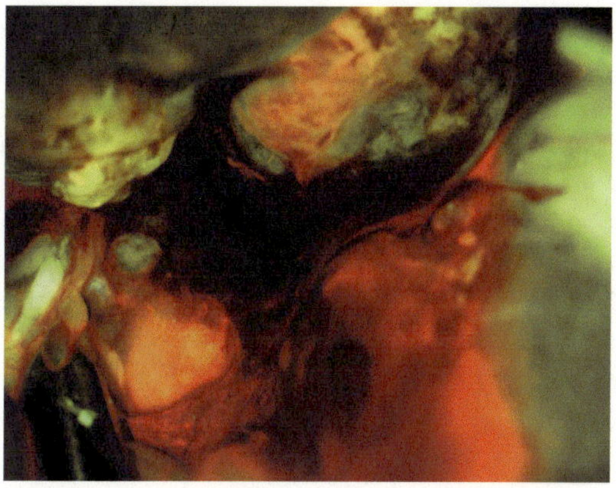

Fig. 10. Uptake of ATX-S10Na(II) in Case 2

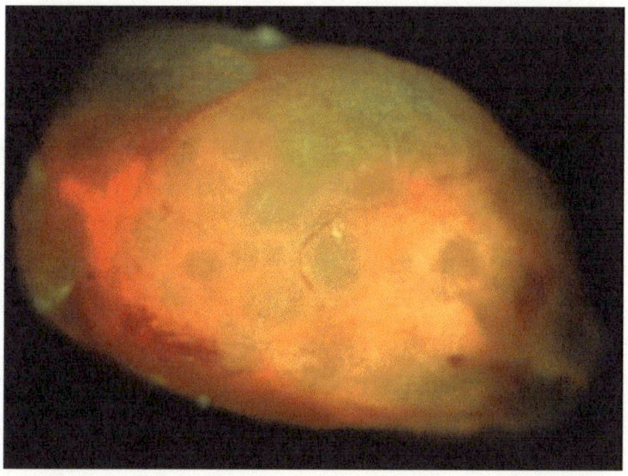

Fig. 11. Isolation of red-emitting Lg-LN stained with ATX-S10Na(II)

In another two examples (Fig. 9 and 10), red-fluorescent ATX-S10Na (II) was incorporated rapidly into afferent lymphatic vessels around the primary lesion, lymphatic network, and flowed first into the Lg-LN. The lymph nodes as well as afferent lymphatic vessels were visualized vividly by this method. Although Case 2 (Fig. 10) was bleeding heavily during experiment, red-emitting LNs were detected easily. After the completion of observation, a red- emitting Lg-LN with metastasis of poorly differentiated adenocarcinoma was harvested and dissected in Case 1 (Fig. 11). The LN continued to emit red fluorescence in the similar degree of intensity at least for 30 minutes. Thus, ATX-S10Na (II) could efficiently visualize lymphatic network around the primary lesion, afferent lymphatic vessel and sentinel node. This method is simple and convenient, since it dose not require radioisotope or gamma probe.

5. Advantage of photosensitizer to tracer

5.1 Visualization of sentinel nodes by strong emission of red fluorescence

ATX-S10Na (II) emits strong red fluorescence with excitation wavelength (Nakajima et al., 1998). As shown in Fig. 7 to 10, the distribution of ATX-S10Na(II) in lymphatic network can be detected clearly and easily by the red fluorescence marking. This photographic visualization allows any observer to clearly identify SNs, and to easily determine the location and orientation of SNs in the orthotopic xenograft animal model. Such direct real-time visualization is not possible using radioactive tracers, which must be measured by scintillation probes or gamma camera (Hayashi et al., 2003; Kim et al., 2004; Kitagawa & Kitajima, 2002; Tanaka et al., 2004). Of note, this novel procedure would be easily conducted in human and in community hospitals without difficulties, because it does not require complicated procedures, special facilities or radioactive substances. Other non-fluorescent dye tracers (Hiratsuka et al., 2001; Ichikura et al., 2002; Hayashi et al., 2003; Miwa et al., 2003; Tanaka et al., 2004) cannot provide such a vivid and colorful contrast. The visual and technical advantage of ATX-S10Na (II) may assist every surgeon to assess SNs accurately in sentinel node navigation surgery, and potentially prevent an oversight for false-negative LNs.

5.2 Rapid incorporation into lymphatic tissues

As a general rule, photosensitizers are systemically administered via a peripheral intravenous route before laser irradiation in photodynamic therapy for various carcinomas. As shown in Fig. 7, however, ATX-S10Na (II) is incorporated rapidly into lymphatic tissues after subserosal injection into the primary tumor. Our study confirmed for the first time that ATX-S10Na (II) is taken up by local lymphatic tissues when it is subserosally injected into the primary tumor lesion (Koyama et al., 2007a). One possible explanation for the phenomenon is that the chemical structure of ATX-S10Na (II) is water-soluble, but not lipid-soluble (Matsumoto et al., 2003; Mori et al., 2000a, 2000b; Nakajima et al., 1992, 1998). Since the uptake of ATX-S10Na (II) into lymphatic system is rapid and its fluorescence can be consistently observed in real time, this approach appears to be useful for shortening the time required for SN biopsy and surgical procedure. Of importance, the ATX-S10Na (II)-guided method is not associated with the "shine-through" phenomenon, whereby the large hot spot at the injection site of radioactive tracers disturbs the detection of SNs around the primary tumor lesion.

5.3 High affinity and specific uptake to tumor cells

ATX-S10Na (II) is a high affinity molecule for tumor cells. Its preferential uptake in target tumor cells results in selective accumulations in tumor tissues, indicating that the tumor-specificity of photodynamic therapy depends largely on the oncotropic properties of photosensitizers (Fisher et al., 1995; Kvam et al., 1990; Matsumoto et al., 2003; Mori et al., 2000a, 2000b; Nakajima et al., 1992, 1998; Sharman et al., 1999). As shown in Fig. 8, ATX-S10Na (II) can be taken up by LNs that are involved with tumor metastases. However, the precise mechanisms of tumor-specific uptake of ATX-S10Na (II) remain unclear. It is proposed that ATX-S10 Na (II) is incorporated into tumor cells by fluid phase endocytosis, receptor-mediated endocytosis, or orphan transporters (Mori et al., 2000b). Alternatively, another possible mechanism is that lymphatic flow is delayed or altered in LNs filled with metastatic tumor cells, resulting in preferential retention of ATX-S10Na (II) in such LNs. In our previous study, the presence of tumor metastases in LNs was assessed by RT-PCR of human β-actin (Koyama et al., 2007a). To our surprise, human β-actin was positive in all LNs located downstream of human-β-actin-positive Lg-LN that was regarded as SN. In contrast, LNs located downstream of human-β-actin-negative Lg-LN (SN) were negative for human β-actin. In addition, all human-β-actin-positive Lg-LNs (SNs) were red nodes, whereas all non-red Lg-LNs (non-SNs) were human β-actin-negative. Considering the higher positive rates by RT-PCR assay than conventional histopathological examination (Bilchik et al., 2001; Kitagawa & Kitajima, 2002; Maruyama et al., 1999; Natsugoe, et al., 1998; Noura et al., 2002), these results showed high sensitivity and specificity of the ATX-S10Na (II)-guided method for the detection of SNs. Because micrometastasis occurs frequently in gastric carcinoma, the system using ATXS10Na(II) may be a novel technology to detect micrometastases with high sensitivity, resulting in reduction of false-negative LNs.

5.4 Little toxicity in human

No obvious toxicity was observed in rats that were injected locally with ATX-S10Na(II) at a dose of 1.3–2.5 mg/kg in our study (Koyama et al., 2007a). This dosage is much smaller than that of systemic administration given intravenously at a dose of 5–25 mg/kg, which caused little, if any, toxicity *in vivo* (Matsumoto et al., 2003; Mori et al., 2000a; Nakajima et al., 1992, 1998). Since ATX-S10Na(II) is a hydrophilic photosensitizer with a low-molecular weight, its clearance from tissues and body (within 24 hours) is much faster than that of the first generation photosensitizers. Therefore, it has substantially less adverse effects (Matsumoto et al., 2003; Mori et al., 2000a; Nakajima et al., 1992; Nakajima et al., 1998). We acknowledge that our studies were conducted in an orthotopic xenograft rat model (Koyama et al, 2007a, 2007b), in which the structure and anatomy of the regional lymphatic network may be different from those of human system (Ichikura et al., 2002; Miwa et al., 2003). Alternatively, the rat model may not be comparable to early gastric carcinoma in humans, for which sentinel node navigation surgery is more suitable (Hiratsuka et al., 2001; Isozaki et al., 2004). Clear visualization of lymphatic system by ATX-S10Na (II) may be only true of the animal model. However, our studies do demonstrate the potential usefulness of ATX-S10Na(II) as a tracer of SNs by assessing tumor metastases with RT-PCR (Koyama et al., 2007a, 2007b). In 25 out of 27 rats, Lg-LN (SN) was identified as a red node, and most of these Lg-LNs (SNs) were positive for human β-actin, which was an indication of tumor metastasis. Of interest, ATX-S10Na(II) was incorporated into the hepatic LN (SN), but not into the Lg-LN (non-SN) in two out of 27 rats, and human β-actin was positive only in the hepatic LN (SN), but not in the Lg-LN (non-SN) in these rats. These findings support the notion that SN is the first LN to receive lymphatic drainage and tumor cells from a primary tumor, and ATX-S10Na(II) is useful for the detection of SNs.

6. Other dye tracers and comparison with ATX-S10Na(II)

Patent blue violet (Hayashi et al., 2003; Karube et al., 2004; Miwa et al., 2003; Simsa et al., 2003), isosulfan blue (Hundley et al., 2002; Isozaki et al., 2004; Lee et al., 2005; Osaka et al., 2004; Ryu et al., 2003; Song t al., 2004) and indocyanine green (ICG) (Hiratsuka et al., 2001; Ichikura et al., 2002; Nimura et al., 2004) have been used as vital dye tracers for the detection of SNs in gastric carcinoma. The detection rates of SNs were 72–96%, 91–100% and 99–100%, respectively. These favorable results must be carefully interpreted because SN mapping is dependent on the technical learning curve and skills of the surgeon (Ichikura et al., 2002; Simsa et al., 2003; Nimura et al., 2004). The sensitivity was 77–90%, 46–100% and 64–90%, respectively, suggesting that non-SNs could contain tumor cell metastases. In most of these reports, the presence of metastasis in LNs was determined by conventional haematoxylin and eosin staining. False-negative rates may increase when more sensitive methods such as multiple sectioning, immunohistochemical staining or RT–PCR technique are used.

Some biomedical imaging techniques use the characteristic feature of ICG; this dye absorbs infrared rays, which enhances its visibility (Flower & Hochheimer, 1976; Kohso et al., 1990). Enhanced visualization of ICG by using a near-infrared endoscopy substantially improves the rate of SN detection in patients with gastric carcinoma, compared with the use of ICG alone (Nimura et al., 2004). Interestingly, SNs illuminated with a near-infrared endoscope are clear enough to be identified by all observers, whereas SNs stained by ICG alone are not always visible to all investigators. As a result, the ICG-guided method combined with a near- infrared endoscope was reported to increase the sensitivity significantly from 64% of patients and 50% of LNs to 100% and 100%, respectively (Nimura et al., 2004). The combination method appears to be a promising approach for biomedical imaging in living tissue.

As shown in Fig. 7 to 10, the rapid migration of ATX-S10Na (II) along the lymphatic system is clearly visualized and easily identified in real time by the strong red fluorescence. Such visualization is clearer than that of enhanced visualization of ICG with a near-infrared laparoscope (Koyama et al., 2007b). Since a much darker operating room is required to ensure the detection of ICG through a near-infrared endoscopy, it may be difficult to perform other procedures. One explanation for the high-quality visualization of ATX-S10Na (II) is that the excitation wavelength peak (450 ± 40 nm) is completely separate from the emission wavelength peak (667 nm). With the visual advantage of ATX-S10Na (II), SNs would not be missed, and the time required for the surgical procedure may be shortened.

In a comparative study using an orthotopic xenograft rat model, there was no significant difference in the detection rates of SNs, the sensitivity, and the number of stained nodes between ATX-S10Na (II)- and enhanced ICG-guided methods (Koyama et al., 2007b). These results suggest that the ATX-S10Na(II)-guided method is comparable to or possibly superior to the enhanced ICG-guided method. In addition, the number of ICG-stained nodes varies widely, since the number and distribution of stained nodes become larger and wider as the injection dose is increased (Ichikura et al., 2002). In the dual-mapping technique with dye and radioactive tracers, significant differences in distributions are noted between the two tracers (Hayashi et al., 2003; Karube et al., 2004). These findings raise the question of whether dye or radioactive traces flow into the lymphatic system in the same manner as metastatic cancer cells. ATX-S10Na (II) may resolve the issue, because it has a high specificity and affinity for tumor cells (Nakajima et al, 1992, 1998; Mori et al., 2000b). In the future, novel fluorescence-based reagents (Kim, S. et al., 2004; Ueno et al., 2005), including photosensi- tizers, will be developed as tracers that improve diagnostic accuracy in sentinel node navigation surgery.

7. Conclusion

A novel system using a hydrophilic photosensitizer ATX-S10Na (II) in combination with a fluorescence spectrolaparoscope is useful for the detection of cancer-containing sentinel nodes in an orthotopic xenograft animal model of human gastric carcinoma. ATX-S10Na (II) would serve as a novel tracer in sentinel node navigation surgery. This system has great potential application for the decision of minimally invasive surgery without radical extensive regional lymphadenectomy in early gastric carcinoma. A comparative study of ATX-S10Na (II) versus other dye tracers will determine whether the red-fluorescent tracer system is useful for lymphatic mapping in sentinel node navigation surgery for patients with early gastric carcinoma.

8. References

Bilchik, A.J.; Saha, S.; Wiese, D; Stonecypher, J.A.; Wood, T.F.; Sostrin, S.; Turner, R.R.; Wang, H.J.; Morton, D.L.; Hoon, D.S. (2001). Molecular staging of early colon cancer on the basis of sentinel node analysis: A multicenter phase II trial. *Journal of Clinical Oncology*, Vol.19, No.4, (February 2001), pp.1128–1136, ISSN 0732-183X

Fisher, A.M.; Murphree, A.L. & Gomer, C.J. (1995). Clinical and preclinical photodynam- ic therapy. *Lasers in Surgery and Medicine*, Vol.17, No.1, pp.2–31, ISSN 0196-8092

Flower, R.W. & Hochheimer. B.F. (1976). Indocyanine green dye fluorescence and infrared absorption choroidal angiography performed simultaneously with fluorescein angiography. *Johns Hopkins Medical Journal*, Vol.138, No.2, (February 1976), pp.33–42, ISSN 0021-7263

Fujihara, T.; Sawada, T.; Hirakawa, K.-Chung, Y.S.; Yashiro, M.; Inoue, T.; Sowa, M. (1998). Establishment of lymph node metastatic model for human gastric cancer in nude mice and analysis of factors associated with metastasis. *Clinical & Experimental Metastasis*, Vol.16, No.4, (May 1998), pp.389–398, ISSN 0262-0898

Hayashi, H.; Ochiai, T.; Mori, M.; Karube, T.; Suzuki, T.; Gunji, Y.; Hori, S.; Akutsu, N.; Matsubara, H.; Shimada, H. (2003). Sentinel lymph node mapping for gastric cancer using a dual procedure with dye- and gamma probe-guided techniques. *Journal of the American College of Surgeons*, Vol.196, No.1, (January 2003), pp.68–74, ISSN 1072-7515

Hiratsuka, M.; Miyashiro, I.; Ishikawa, O.; Furukawa, H.; Motomura, K.; Ohigashi, H.; Kameyama, M.; Sasaki, Y.; Kabuto, T.; Ishiguro, S.; Imaoka, S.; Koyama, H. (2001). Application of sentinel node biopsy to gastric cancer surgery. *Surgery*, Vol.129, No.3, (March 2001), pp.335-340, ISSN 0039- 6060

Hundley, J.C.; Shen, P.; Shiver, S.A.; Geisinger, K.R.; Levine, E.A. (2002). Lymphatic mapping for gastric adenocarci- noma. *American Surgeon*, Vol.68, No.11, (November 2002), pp.931–935, ISSN 0003-1348

Ichikura, T.; Morita, D.; Uchida, T.; Okura, E.; Majima, T.; Ogawa, T.; Mochizuki, H. (2002). Sentinel node concept in gastric carcinoma. *World Journal of Surgery*, Vol.26, No.3, (March 2002), pp.318–322, ISSN 0364-2313

Isozaki, H.; Kimura, T.; Tanaka, N.; Satoh, K.; Matsumoto, S.; Ninomiya, M.; Ohsaki, T.; Mori, M. (2004). An assessment of the feasibility of sentinel lymph node-guided surgery for gastric cancer. *Gastric Cancer*, Vol.7, No.3, pp.149–153

Karube, T.; Ochiai, T.; Shimada, H.; Nikaidou, T.; Hayashi, H. (2004). Detection of sentinel lymph nodes in gastric cancers based on immunohistochemical analysis of micrometastases. *Journal of Surgical Oncology*, Vol.87, No.1, (July 2004), pp.32–38, ISSN 0022-4790

Kim, S.; Lim, Y.T.; Soltesz, E.G.; De Grand, A.M.; Lee, J.; Nakayama, A.; Parker, J.A.; Mihaljevic, T.; Laurence, R.G.; Dor, D.M.; Cohn, L.H.; Bawendi, M.G.; Frangioni, J.V. (2004). Near-infrared fluorescent type II quantum dots for sentinel lymph node maping. *Nature Biotechnology*, Vol.22, No.1, (January 2004), pp.93–97, ISSN 1087-0156

Kim, M.C.; Kim, H.H.; Jung, G.J.; Lee, J.H.; Choi, S.R.; Kang, D.Y.; Roh, M.S.; Jeong, J.S. (2004). Lymphatic mapping and sentinel node biopsy using 99mTc tin colloid in gastric cancer. *Annals of Surgery*, Vol.239, No.3, (March 2004), pp.383–387, ISSN 0003-4932

Kitagawa, Y. & Kitajima, M. (2002). Gastrointestinal cancer and sentinel node navigation surgery. *Journal of Surgical Oncology*, Vol.79, No.3, (March 2002), pp.188–193, ISSN 0022-4790

Kohso, H.; Tatsumi, Y.; Fujino, H.; Tokita, K.; Kodama, T.; Kashima, K.; Kawai, K. (1990). An investigation of an infrared ray electronic endoscope with a laser diode light source. *Endoscopy*, Vol.22, No.5, (September 1990), pp.217–220, ISSN 0013-726X

Koyama, T.; Tsubota, A.; Nariai, K.; Yoshikawa, T.; Mitsunaga, M.; Sumi, M.; Nimura, H.; Yanaga, K.; Yumoto, Y.; Mabashi, Y.; Takahashi, H. (2007a). Detection of sentinel nodes by a novel red-fluorescent dye, ATX-S10Na(II), in an orthotopic xenograft rat model of human gastric carcinoma. *Lasers in Surgery and Medicine*, Vol39. No.1, (January 2007), pp.76–82, ISSN 0196-8092

Koyama, T.; Tsubota, A.; Nariai, K.; Mitsunaga, M.; Yanaga, K.; Takahashi, H. (2007b). Novel biomedical imaging approach for detection of sentinel nodes in an experimental model of gastric cancer. *British Journal of Surgery*, Vol.94, No.8, (August 2007), pp.996-1001, ISSN 0007-1323

Krag, D.; Weaver, D.; Ashikaga, T.; Moffat, F.; Klimberg, V.S.; Shriver, C.; Feldman, S.; Kusminsky, R.; Gadd, M.; Kuhn, J.; Harlow, S.; Beitsch, P. (1998). The sentinel node in breast cancer—a multicenter validation study. *New England Journal of Medicine*, Vol.339, No.14, (October 1998), pp.941–946, ISSN 0028-4793

Kvam, E., Stokke, T. & Moan, J. (1990). The lengths of DNA fragments light-induced in the presence of a photosensitizer localized at the nuclear membrane of human cells. *Biochimica et Biophysica Acta*, Vol.1049, No.1, (May 1990), pp.33–37, ISSN 0006-3002

Lee, J.H.; Ryu, K.W.; Kim, C.G.; Kim, S.K.; Choi, I.J.; Kim, Y.W.; Chang, H.J.; Bae, J.M.; Hong, E.K. (2005). Comparative study of the subserosal *versus* submucosal dye injection method for sentinel node biopsy in gastric cancer. *European Journal of Surgical Oncology*, Vol.31, No.9, (November 2005), pp.965–968, ISSN 0748-7983

Maruyama, K.; Sasako, M.; Kinoshita, T.; Sano, T.; Katai, H. (1999). Can sentinel node biopsy indicate rational extent of lymphadenectomy in gastric cancer surgery? Fundamental and new information on lymph-node dissection. *Langenbeck's Archives of Surgery*, Vol. 384, No.2, (April 1999), pp.149–157, ISSN 1435-2443

Masumoto, K.; Yamada, I.; Tanaka, H.; Fujise, Y.; Hashimoto, K. (2003). Tissue distribution of a new photosensitizer ATX-S10Na (II) and effect of a diode laser (670 nm) in photody- namic therapy. *Lasers in Medical Science*, Vol.18, No.3, pp.134–138, ISSN 0268-8921

Miwa, K.; Kinami, S.; Taniguchi, K.; Fushida, S.; Fujimura, T.; Nonomura, A. (2003). Mapping sentinel nodes in patients with early stage gastric carcinoma. *British Journal of Surgery*, Vol.90, No.2, (February 2003), pp.178–182, ISSN 0007-1323

Mori, M.; Sakata, I.; Hirano, T.; Obana, A.; Nakajima, S.; Hikida, M.; Kumagai, T. (2000a). Photodynamic therapy for experimental tumors using ATX-S10 (Na), a hydrophilic chlorin photosensitizer, and diode laser. *Japanese Journal of Cancer Research*, Vol.91, No.7, (July 2000), pp.753–759, ISSN 0910-5050

Mori, M.; Kuroda, T.; Obana, A.; Sakata, I.; Hirano, T.; Nakajima, S.; Hikida, M.; Kumagai, T. (2000b). In vitro plasma protein binding and cellu- lar uptake of ATX-S10 (Na), a hydrophilic chlorine photosensitizer. *Japanese Journal of Cancer Research*, Vol.91, No.8, (August 2000), pp.845–852, ISSN 0910-5050

Morton, D.L.; Wen, D.R.; Wong, J.H.; Economou, J.S.; Cagle, L.A.; Storm, F.K.; Foshag, L.J.; Cochran, A.J. (1992). Technical details of intraoperative lymphatic mapping for early stage melanoma. *Archives of Surgery*, Vol.127, No.4, (November 1991), pp.392–399, ISSN 0004-0010

Nakajima, S.; Sakata, I.; Takemura, T.; Maeda, T.; Hayashi, H.; Kubo, Y.; Samejima, N.; Koshimizu, K. (1992). Tumor localizing and photosensitiza- tion of photo-chlorin ATX-S10, In: *Photodynamic therapy and biomedical lasers*, Spinelli, P.; Fante, D.M.; Marchesini, R. (Ed.), 531–534, Elsevier Science, Amsterdam

Nakajima, S.; Sakata, I.; Hirano, T.; Takemura, T. (1998). Therapeutic effect of interstitial photody- namic therapy using ATX-S10 (Na) and a diode laser on radio-resistant SCCVII tumors of C3H/He mice. *Anti-cancer Drugs*, Vol.9, No.6, (July 1998), pp.539–543, ISSN 0959-4973

Natsugoe, S.; Mueller, J.; Stein, H.J.; Feith, M.; Hofler, H.; Siewert, J.R. (1998). Micrometastasis and tumor cell microin- volvement of lymph nodes from esophageal squamous cell carcinoma: Frequency, associated tumor characteristics, and impact on prognosis. *Cancer*, Vol. 83, No.5, (September 1998), pp.858–866, ISSN 0008-543X

Nimura, H.; Narimiya, N.; Mitsumori, N.; Yamazaki, Y.; Yanaga, K.; Urashima, M. (2004). Infrared ray electronic endoscopy combined with indocyanine green injection for detection of sentinel nodes of patients with gastric cancer. *British Journal of Surgery*, Vol.91, No.5, (May 2004), pp.575–579, ISSN 0007-1323

Noura, S., Yamamoto, H., Ohnishi, T.; Masuda, N.; Matsumoto, T.; Takayama, O.; Fukunaga, H.; Miyake, Y.; Ikenaga, M.; Ikeda, M.; Sekimoto, M.; Matsuura, N.; Monden, M. (2002). Comparative detection of lymph node micrometastases of stage II colorectal cancer by reverse transcriptase polymerase chain reaction and immunohistochem- istry. *Journal of Clinical Oncology*, Vol.20, No. 20, (October 2002), pp.4232–4241, ISSN 0732-183X

Osaka, H.; Yashiro, M.; Sawada, T.; Katsuragi, K.; Hirakawa, K. (2004). Is a lymph node detected by the dye-guided method a true sentinel node in gastric cancer? *Clinical Cancer Research*, Vol.10, No.20, (October 2004), pp.6912–6918, ISSN 1078-0432

Ryu, K.W.; Lee, J.H.; Kim, H.S.; Kim, Y.W.; Choi, I.J.; Bae, J.M.. (2003). Prediction of lymph nodes metastasis by sentinel node biopsy in gastric cancer. *European Journal of Surgical Oncology*, Vol.29, No.10, (December 2003), pp.895–899, ISSN 0748-7983

Sharman, W.M.; Allen, C.M. & van Lier, J.E. (1999). Photodynamic therapeutics: basic principles and clinical applications. *Drug Discovery Today*, Vol.4, No.11, (November 1999), pp.507–517, ISSN 1359-6446

Simsa, J.; Hoch, J.; Leffler, J.; Schwarz, J.; Pospisil, R.; Vajtrova, R. (2003). Sentinel node biopsy in gastric cancer: preliminary results. *Acta Chirurgica Belgica*, Vol.103, No.3, (June 2003), pp.270–273, ISSN 0001-5458

Sobin, L.H. (2003). TNM, sixth edition: New developments in general concepts and rules. *Seminars in Surgical Oncology*, Vol.21, No.1, (August 2003), pp.19–22, ISSN 1098-2388

Song, X; Wang, L.; Chen, W.; Pan, T.; Zhu, H.; Xu, J.; Jin, M.; Finley, R.K.; Wu, J. (2004). Lymphatic mapping and sentinel node biopsy in gastric cancer. *American Journal of Surgery* Vol.187, No.2, (February 2004), pp.270–273, ISSN 0002-9610

Tanaka, K., Tonouchi, H., Kobayashi, M.; Konishi, N.; Ohmori, Y.; Mohri, Y.; Kusunoki, M. (2004). Laparoscopically assisted total gastrectomy with sentinel node biopsy for early gastric cancer: Preliminary results. *American Surgeon,* Vol.70, No.11, (November 2004), pp.976–981, ISSN 0003-1348

Ueno, H.; Hihara, J.; Shimizu, K.; Osaki, A.; Yamashita, Y.; Yoshida, K.; Toge, T. (2005). Experimental study on fluorescent microspheres as a tracer for sentinel node detection. *Anticancer Research,* Vol.25, No.2A, (March-April 2005), pp.821–825, ISSN 0250-7005

van der Veen, H.; Hoekstra, O.S.; Paul, M.A.; Cuesta, M.A.; Meijer, S. (1994). Gamma probe-guided sentinel node biopsy to select patients with melanoma for lymphadenectomy. *British Journal of Surgery,* Vol.81, No.12, (December 1994), pp.1769–1770, ISSN 0007-1323

Veronesi, U.; Paganelli, G.; Galimberti, V.; Viale, G.; Zurrida, S.; Bedoni, M.; Costa, A.; de Cicco, C.; Geraghty, J.G.; Luini, A.; Sacchini, V.; Veronesi, P. (1997). Sentinel-node biopsy to avoid axillary dissection in breast cancer with clinically negative lymph-nodes. *Lancet,* Vol.349, No.9069, (June 1997), pp.1864–1867, ISSN 0140-6736

Part 2

Surgery

5

Laparoscopic Surgery for Gastric Cancer

Kyo Young Song and Jung Ho Shim
Division of Gastrointestinal Surgery, Department of Surgery, Minimal Access and Robotic Surgery Center, Seoul St. Mary's Hospital, College of Medicine, The Catholic University of Korea, Seoul, Republic of Korea

1. Introduction

Even though an overall incidence of the gastric cancer has been declined it remains as the second leading cause of cancer-related deaths world widely with the highest incidence in Korea and Japan. [1]

Over the past decade, however, the overall survival rate of patients with gastric cancer has been increased. This increased survival resulted from not only the early detection with an intensive surveillance in accordance of the development of an endoscopy but also the aggressive surgery approaches including an extensive lymph node dissection; combined with a resection of adjacent organs, if indicated. Additionally the improved perioperative management on the patients has improved the survival. [2]

Since the first case of a laparoscopy-assisted gastrectomy was reported by Kitano et al. in 1994, [3] the number of patients underwent laparoscopic gastrectomy for early gastric cancer (EGC) has been increased rapidly especially in Korea and Japan, where there is a high incidence of EGC. According to survey by the Korean Gastric Cancer Association in 2009, the number of gastric cancer operations performed laparoscopically has surprisingly increased (Fig. 1).

The technical innovations in laparoscopic instrument and the advances in the surgical techniques have allowed for a widespread acceptance of a laparoscopic surgery in gastric cancer management. The Advantages of the laparoscopic gastrectomy over the conventional open surgery include a reduced postoperative pain, an enhanced recovery, a shorter hospital stay, and a better cosmesis. [4,5] Although there is a high level of an evidence to support short-term efficacy of a laparoscopic gastrectomy for EGC, still the long term results accounts on the patients' survival are still infrequent. The technical feasibility of the laparoscopic radical lymphadenectomy must need to be proven in the long-term, and the oncologic concerns involved in laparoscopic gastrectomy such as the oncological effects of a pneumoperitoneum, must still be resolved. A prospective multi-center randomized clinical trial has started to assess the short- and long-term outcomes of laparoscopic gastrectomy for early stage gastric cancer (KLASS trial, Korean Laparoscopic Gastro-intestinal Surgery Study Group) on March 2005.

This review will summarize the current status for laparoscopic surgery for gastric cancer, ongoing controversies on the clinical trial, and the future perspectives of the minimally invasive treatment.

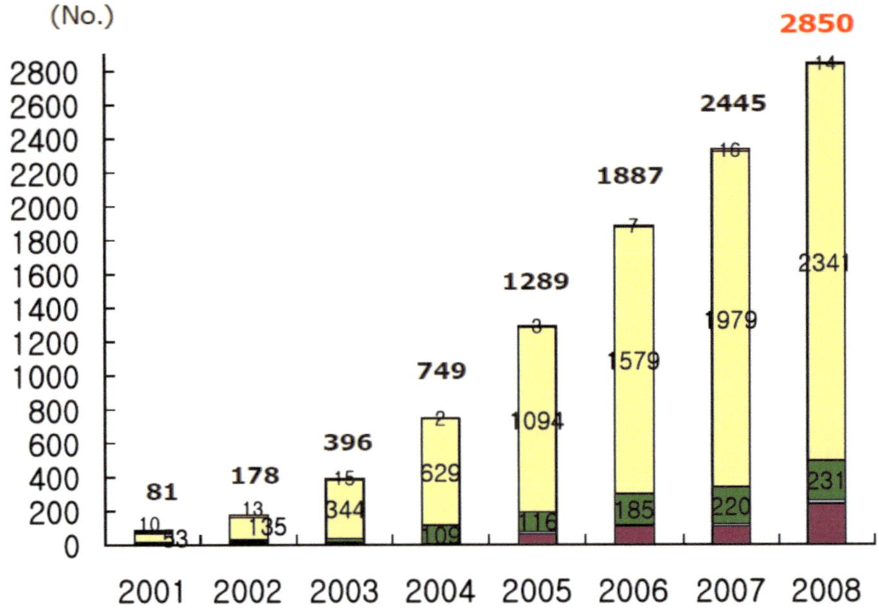

Fig. 1. Annual number of laparoscopic procedures performed for gastric adenocarcinoma in Korea. Orange bar, wedge resection; yellow bar, distal gastrectomy; green bar, total gastrectomy; sky blue bar, gastrojejunostomy; purple bar, other procedures

2. History and the current status of laparoscopic surgery for gastric cancer

The history of laparoscopic gastric surgery dates from 1992, when Peter Goh of Singapore performed the first entirely laparoscopic Billroth II distal gastrectomy on a patient affected with chronic gastric ulcer. [6] The first laparoscopic wedge resection for gastric cancer was carried out by Ohgami et al. [7] They used a T-fastener and performed an intragastric mucosal resection for a patient with EGC in 1992. (Fig. 2) And Ohashi et al. attempted the intragastric mucosal resection (IGMR) for EGC of the stomach located at the posterior wall for the first time [8]. The aim of both procedures was to minimize the extent of gastric resection for the treatment of a malignant disease with a low risk of lymph node metastasis, therefore to reduce the accompanying physiologic side effects by the standard gastrectomy.

In June 1993, J.S. Azagra performed their first laparoscopic gastrectomy for gastric cancer. [9] Kitano et al. had reported the first laparoscopy-assisted distal gastrectomy (LADG) with D1+α lymph node dissection for EGC in 1994. Since then, various types of laparoscopic gastric surgery have been successfully performed using laparoscopy. Recent advances in techniques for performing the lymph node dissection and the development of new instrumentations, such as stapling devices and ultrasonic devices, have made it possible to perform almost all the procedures in gastrectomy with lymphadenectomy laparoscopically which comparable to the open conventional surgery. Function-preserving surgery, such as pylorus preserving surgery, proximal gastrectomy, and segmental gastrectomy has been also successfully performed by laparoscopy.

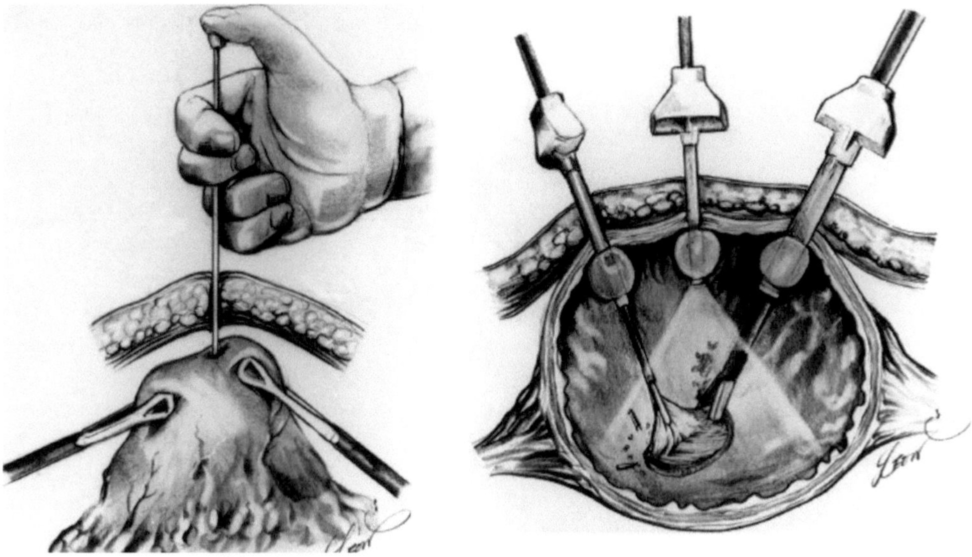

Source : World J Surg 1999;23:187-193. [7]

Fig. 2. Lesion lifting technique with T-fastener originally reported by Ohgami et al. in 1992.

Recently, these laparoscopic gastrectomies have been increased remarkably in Japan and Korea. A national Japanese survey showed that more than 4500 patients with gastric cancer underwent laparoscopic gastrectomy in 2007. [10] Although LADG was first reported as a minimally invasive surgery for EGC, some aggressive surgeons successfully performed extended (D2) lymph node dissection on patient so that LADG can be used to treat AGC. [11,12] There are surgeons who are now trying to expand the indications of laparoscopy-assisted gastrectomy to the treatment options for an advanced gastric cancer. In 1999, Uyama et al. [13] reported the result of LADG with D2 lymph node dissection for advanced cancer. With the exception of early reports, the retrieved number of lymph nodes in laparoscopic surgery for advanced gastric cancer has been reported as equivalent to that in open surgery. Korean surgeons could acquire advanced-laparoscopic skills for gastrectomy by maintaining the exchange fellowship program and the clinical researches with the expert in Japan. Considering that the majority of gastric cancer patients in Korea are managed by a limited number of experts at high-volume centers, it was easy for the Korean surgeons to catch up with high level of the proficiency. The wide acceptance and the development of laparoscopic surgery for malignant gastric disease in the West have been increased slowly. Laparoscopy-assisted distal, subtotal, or total gastrectomy for early and advanced gastric cancer is now emerging in the West with progressive acceptance among various groups, although this upward trend has been slowed by the difference in natural history of gastric adenocarcinoma in the East compared with the West. [14]

3. Optimal extent of lymph node dissection for gastric cancer

The extent of lymph node dissection for gastric cancer has consistently been a subject of debate world widely. Three types of laparoscopic lymph node dissection are performed (Table 1): perigastric lymph node dissection (D1 + α), additional lymph node dissection along the common hepatic artery (D1 + β), and extended lymph node dissection covered for non-regional lymph nodes. (D2). [15]

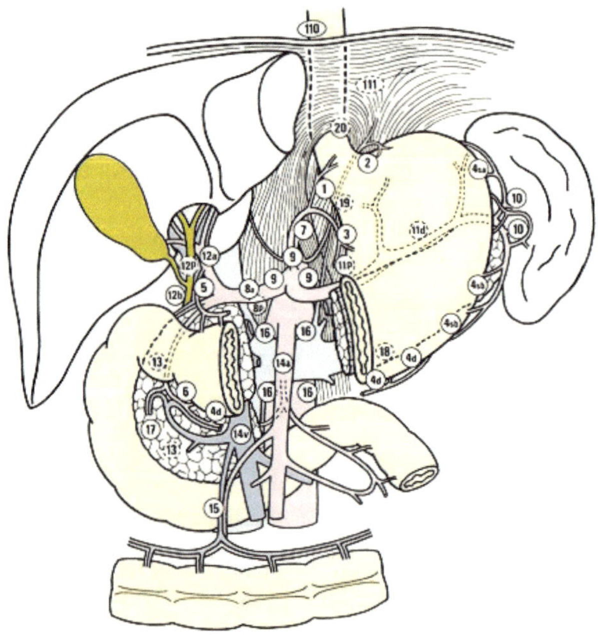

Source: Japanese Gastric Cancer Association. Japanese Classification of Gastric Carcinoma; 2nd English Edition. [15]

Fig. 3. Perigastric regional lymph node stations.

D2 dissection has been a standard procedure in Japan and Korea although it was not based on the clinical trial. Two European randomized trials comparing D2 with D1 dissection was failed to show a survival benefit of D2 dissection, which was resulted in high rate of a postoperative mortality. [16, 17] However, the survival benefit in these trials seems to be biased on the technical factors and the patients' selection factors which was resulted in the high rate of postoperative complications and high operative mortality rates. A report from the retrospective analyses series have shown superior stage-by-stage survival rates when compared with data from other countries in which D2 dissection is not a standard procedure. Extended lymph node dissection remains a standard of care in the Far East and also in Western specialized units where it can be conducted safely. [18]

D0 : No dissection or incomplete dissection of the Group 1 nodes
D1 : Dissection of all the Group 1 nodes
D2 : Dissection of all the Group 1 and Group 2 nodes
D3 : Dissection of all the Group 1, Group 2 and Group 3 nodes

Table 1. Definition of lymph node dissection(D)

With the advances of laparoscopic technique in gastric cancer surgery, the standard surgical procedure for EGC has been discussed. Initially, laparoscopic gastrectomy was indicated only for EGC patients with a low risk of lymph node metastasis. The Japanese Gastric

Cancer Association proposed clinical guidelines for the treatment of gastric cancer in 2001. Based on those recommendations, laparoscopic gastrectomy (LG) is recommended for gastric cancer patients with a preoperative stage Ia (cT1N0M0) diagnosis. Although a number of institutes adhere to the guideline, laparoscopic gastrectomy has also been referred to as a pre-established technique that is still under clinical investigation due to the uncertain quality of lymph node dissection and the lack of proof based on long term follow-up data. [15]

Yasuda et al. [19] recommended D1 + α lymph node dissection for submucosal cancer measured 1–4 cm in diameter based on pathologic report. Hyung et al. [20] proposed D2 lymph node dissection for a differentiated submucosal cancer more than 2.5 cm in diameter and for undifferentiated submucosal cancer more than 1.5cm. The Japanese Gastric Cancer Association (JGCA) guidelines have set the optimal lymph node dissection level for EGC. Based on a large nationwide registry data, JGCA defined modified gastrectomies A and B (MG-A, MG-B) for treatment of EGC. MG-A is indicated for clinically mucosal cancer or small (< 1.5cm) differentiated-type submucosal cancer. And MG-A proposed dissecting the perigastric nodes and those along the left gastric artery are resected (D1 + No. 7). MG-B is indicated for the submucosal cancers and small (< 2 cm) EGC with clinical N1 disease. In this procedure, the nodes along the hepatic artery (No. 8a) and celiac artery (No. 9) should be resected in addition to those of MG-A. In other EGCs (N1 and > 2 cm, or N2), D2 standard gastrectomy is recommended. In total gastrectomy for proximal EGC, the spleen may be preserved because the lymph nodes metastases in the splenic hilar nodes are extremely rare in EGC.

4. Procedure of laparoscopy assisted distal gastrectomy

Under a pneumoperitoneum at a pressure of 12 mmHg, the greater omentum is divided proximally about 4 to 5 cm from the gastroepiploic arcade toward the lower pole of the spleen using laparoscopic ultrasonic shears (Harmonic Scalpel; Ethicon Endo-Surgery, Cincinnati,OH, USA). For the patients with gastric cancer located in the middle third of the stomach, the roots of left gastroepiploic vessels are exposed and divided with double clipping at their origin from the splenic artery. For the patients with gastric cancer located in the lower third of the stomach, the superior mesenteric vein is exposed with an aid of ultrasonic shears and hooks, and fatty tissue with small lymph nodes (No. 14v) is cleared (Fig. 4). The right gastroepiploic vein is divided at the level of the pancreas border, and the right gastroepiploic artery is then divided at its roots by double clipping after No. 4sb lymph nodes are divided away from the greater curvature. After the right gastric artery have been exposed and divided at its origin by double clipping, the duodenum is transected 1 cm distal to the pylorus via an endoscopic stapler (Endocutter 45 staple; Ethicon, Endo-Surgery, Cincinnati,OH, USA). The lymph nodes with fatty tissue along the hepatic artery (No. 12a), the anterosuperior aspect of common hepatic artery (No. 8a), the celiac axis (No. 9), and the proximal splenic artery (No. 11p) are dissected along each artery using an ultrasonic dissector and a hook-type monopolar bovie. The left gastric vein is divided, and the root of the left gastric artery was exposed and divided with double clipping, thereby allowing dissection of the left gastric artery lymph nodes (No. 7). The perigastric lymph nodes are dissected along the upper lesser curvature up to the esophagogastric junction. The mobilized stomach is then pulled out through this minilaparotomy. After removing the specimens, Billroth I gastroduodenostomy using a circular stapler (Proximate CDH 25;

Ethicon Endo-Surgery, Cincinnati, OH, USA) or Billroth II gastrojejunostomy by hand sewing are performed. [21]

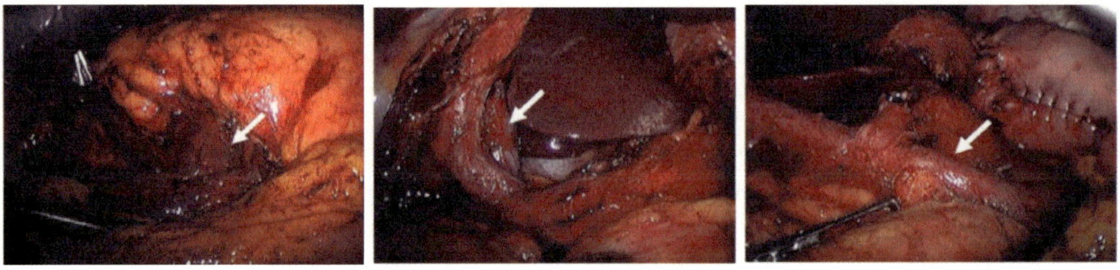

Fig. 4. Intraoperative view after completion of the laparoscopic lymph node dissection White arrow indicates the superior mesenteric vein (a), the portal vein (b), and the splenic artery (c).

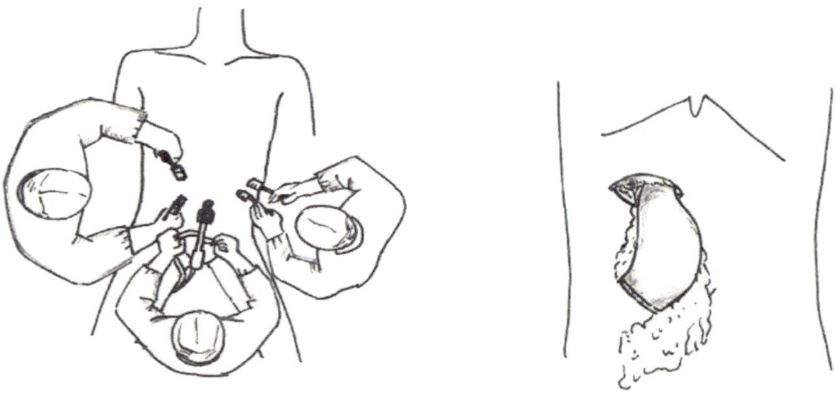

Fig. 5. Laparoscopy assisted distal gastrectomy. The position of patients and operating team are different between theinstitutions. The author prefer to use semi-lithotomy position and operator stands at patient's right side.(left) After full mobilization of stomach and resection of duodenum, half to two thirds of stomach is resected and gastroduodenal anastomosis is followed.(right)

5. Function preserving laparoscopic surgery

To improve the quality of life after gastrectomy, various types of the function-preserving surgery were designed to perform in the laparoscopic era. The proximal gastrectomy, the pylorus preserving gastrectomy, or the vagus nerve preserved gastrectomy is the good examples for the function-preserving gastrectomies. Laparoscopic proximal gastrectomy has performed for EGC located in the proximal third of the stomach. [22] Pylorus-preserving gastrectomy (PPG) was originally indicated as a treatment option for gastric ulcers, but is now applied for patients with EGC located in the distal two-thirds of the stomach. The distal 2/3 of the stomach is resected but approximately 2 cm from a pyloric cuff should be preserved in this procedure. The hepatic and pyloric branches of the vagus nerve are also should be preserved. All the regional lymph nodes, except the suprapyloric nodes (No. 5) can be dissected as in the standard D2 operation. PPG is currently indicated for EGC, located at the mid third of the stomach, which the nodal metastasis to No. 5 is extremely uncommon. The incidence of postgastrectomy dumping syndrome and the risk of the stone formation in a gall bladder (GB) appears to be decreased, and the tendency of the body weight recovery is acceptable compared to that of Billroth I reconstruction. [23] Following the establishment of laparoscopy-assisted PPG (LAPPG), this procedure has been used in many institutions. [24]

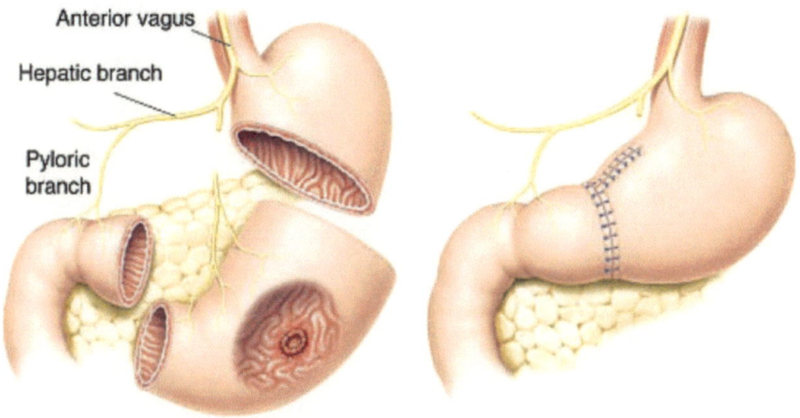

Fig. 6. Pylorus preserving gastrectomy. The pyloric cuff, 2-3 cm from the pyloric ring, is preserved together with the hepatic and pyloric branch of the anterior vagal trunk. Source: Scand J Surg. 2006; 95(4):249-255. [25]

6. Short-term outcomes after laparoscopic gastrectomy

Analysis of data from various retrospective case series almost invariably revealed show that laparoscopic gastrectomy can now be performed safely with less amount of the blood loss, although it usually requires a little bit longer operating time. (Table 2)
Only six RCTs that compared LADG to ODG have been published (Table 3). Kitano et al. [26] had reported no difference in the morbidity and mortality rates between 14 LADG and 14 ODG for EGC. An RCT by Huscher et al., [27] compared the clinical outcomes of LADG with those of ODG for EGC and AGC showed that the morbidity and mortality rates were almost the same between the two procedures. These results suggest that LADG is technically feasible in patients with gastric cancer. Korean Surgeons performed a multi-institutional, prospective, randomized trial for LADG to assess the short- and long-term outcomes of laparoscopy assisted distal gastrectomy (LADG) for EGC in Korea (Korea Laparoscopic Gastrointestinal Surgery Study Group, KLASS trial). A total of 342 patients were randomized (LADG, 179 patients; ODG, 161 patients). [28] There were no significant intraoperative complications or incidence of open conversion in the LADG group. Early complications occurred in 20 patients (11.6%) in the LADG group and 27 patients (15.08%) in the ODG group, and the late complications occurred in three patients each, (1.74% and 1.67%) among the two groups; there were no statistically significant differences in terms of

complications rates between these two groups. Re-operations were performed in 3 patients in the LADG group; (1) omentectomy was performed because of intra-abdominal bleeding, (2) segmental resection of an afferent loop was performed, and (3)primary repair of an leakage at the anastomotic site was done to control peritonitis. In the ODG group, three patients underwent reoperation because of the anastomotic leakage, the postoperative adhesive ileus, and the wound dehiscence. Mortality occurred in two patients in the LADG group; one patient who died of liver function failure due to the chronic hepatitis B, in combination with multiple organ failure. And the other one who had liver cirrhosis (Child B) and chronic renal failure die of a sudden exacerbation of chronic liver disease and resulted in acute liver failure. Even with the aid of the intensive care, these patients have died in 30 and 31 days postoperatively. The morbidities and mortalities were not statistically different between the two groups ($P > 0.49$).

Study (year)	Country	*n*		Level of L/N dissection	Indication
		LADG	ODG		
Adachi (2000)	Japan	49	53	D1+ α	T1a or T1b
Shimizu (2000)	Japan	21	31	D1+ α	T1a
Yano (2001)	Japan	24	35	D1+ α	T1a or superficial T1b
Migoh (2003)	Japan	10	17	D1+ α	T1a or T1b
Miura (2004)	Japan	89	342	D1,D2	T1a or T1b
Noshiro (2005)	Japan	37	31	D2	T1 or T2N0
Tanimura (2005)	Japan	235	200	D2	T1 or T2aN0
Mochiki (2005)	Japan	89	60	D1+β	T1N0
Naka (2005)	Japan	20	22	D1+ β	T1N0
Kim (2005)	Korea	16	16	D2	T1a or T1b
Kim (2005)	Korea	71	76	D1+ α, β, D2	T1aN0
Cho (2006)	Korea	38	35	D1+ β, D2	T1N0-1, T2N0
Ikenaga (2006)	Japan	47	33	D1+ β	T1a
Lee (2006)	Korea	136	120	D1+ β	T1a
Shin (2007)	Korea	80	97	D1+ β	T1a or T1b
Song (2007)	Korea	44	31	D2	T1a or T1b

Table 2. Retrospective studies for comparing open versus laparoscopic gastrectomy

Kodera et al. [29] performed meta-analyses of the following parameters based on randomized trials only, of which there are currently 6 comparing laparoscopy-assisted distal gastrectomy with open distal gastrectomy; the estimated blood loss, the operating time, the number of lymph nodes retrieved, the morbidity and mortality. Quality of the randomized trials would have to be considered as rather mixed, as the KLASS trial is the only multicenter trial with a large sample size. Most notably, the estimated blood loss was reduced at the cost of longer operating time. Surgical complications seemed to be considerably less common with the laparoscopic approach by the meta-analysis, although

Authors	Year	Country	Number of patients	
			LADG	ODG
Kitano	2002	Japan	14	14
Lee	2005	Korea	24	23
Hayashi	2005	Japan	14	14
Huscher	2005	Italy	30	29
Kim YW	2008	Korea	82	82
Kim HH	2010	Korea	179	161

Table 3. Characteristics of the 6 randomized clinical trials

statistical significance had been lacking in the individual studies. A surprisingly high morbidity for open surgery in a trial by Lee and colleagues [30] was thought to be caused by the inclusion of pulmonary complications. The reason that it was so unusually frequent is unknown, but might be attributed to inadequate criteria for reporting such events, it could have occurred by chances, or the limited number of cohort size of the individual trials. In-hospital mortality was acceptable ranges and minimized in all of the studies, as has been shown in other retrospective case series of both laparoscopic and open surgery in the Far East. On the other hand, the quality of lymphadenectomy in terms of the number of the retrieved lymph nodes highly favored open surgery. This result conflicts with earlier findings by some single-institutional retrospective studies, but a meta-analysis of randomized trials only should be regarded as less biased. Whether the difference in retrieval translates into difference in long-term survival remains unknown.

7. Long-term outcomes after laparoscopic gastrectomy

There was a report of an odd recurrence among patients operated on during the 1990s that casts doubt about the oncologic feasibility of laparoscopic surgery for gastric cancer when the surgical technique is im-mature. [31] However, long-term outcomes of the same case series as a whole were excellent. Lee et al. [32] reported the long term oncologic outcomes from laparoscopic gastrectomy 601 cases. At a median follow-up time of 35.9 months (range 3 to 113 months), cancer recurrence occurred in 15 patients and metachronous gastric remnant cancer was detected in 6 patients. The 5-year overall and disease-free survival rates were 94.2% and 89.9%, respectively, for stage IA tumors, 87.4% and 82.7% for stage IB, 80.8% and 70.7% for stage IIA, and 69.6% and 63.1% for stage IIB.

A more extensive retrospective analysis of patients by expert laparoscopic surgeons also revealed excellent outcomes. Japanese Laparoscopic Surgery Study Group analyzed 1,185 cases of laparoscopy-assisted distal gastrectomy. [33] At a median follow-up time of 36 months, estimated 5-year disease-free survival rates were 99.8% for stage IA, 98.7% for stage IB, and 85.7% for stage II. Similarly, the excellent retrospective data suggested the non-inferiority of the laparoscopic approach to treat early-stage cancer have been reported from the KLASS group. [34] A retrospective multicenter study was performed using data from a cohort of 1,485 patients who had undergone laparoscopy-assisted gastrectomy for gastric cancer at ten institutions from 1998 to 2005. The 5-year overall survival of 1,417 patients was 95.5%, and disease-free survival was 94.1%. Fifty of 1,417 patients (3.5%) had recurrences. Incidence of recurrence was 1.6% (19/1186) in early gastric cancer and 13.4% (31/231) in advanced gastric cancer.

One Italian prospective, randomized clinical trial with a total of 59 patients was reported in 2005. [35] Twenty-nine (49.1%) patients were randomized to undergo open subtotal gastrectomy (OG), while 30 (50.9%) patients were randomized to the laparoscopic group (LG). Five-year overall and disease-free survival rates were 55.7% and 54.8% and 58.9% and 57.3% in the OG and the LG, respectively.
These encouraging data prompted several experienced investigators in Japan and Korea to extend the indication for laparoscopic approach to more advanced gastric cancers. Also, large multicenter clinical trial had been conducted and studied the long term oncologic outcomes in gastric cancer looked forward to the final results.

8. Ongoing prospective clinical trials

Randomized trials to prove the oncologic feasibility and safety of laparoscopic surgery as well as to confirm its clinical benefits are mandatory. Korean surgeons who had much larger patient cohorts were actively to launch a phase III trial. After an initial attempt, they launched the KLASS group trial (NCT00452751), a large-scale multi-institutional trial. The Japanese Gastric Cancer Treatment Guidelines discreetly selected early-stage cancer (T1N0, T1N1 or T2 (MP)-T3 (SS) N0) as tentative targets of laparoscopic surgery. The Koreans referred to these guidelines and recruited only patients with preoperative diagnosis of stage I disease in the trial. They identified comorbidity of the patients and lack of experience on the side of surgeons as risk factors for complications in their preparatory retrospective analysis, [36] and only surgeons with experience of more than 50 laparoscopic gastrectomy procedures were invited to participate in the phase III trial. The first convincing evidence of oncologic outcomes of the laparoscopic procedure will be available in the near future from Korea.
More recently, the Japan Clinical Oncology Group (JCOG) began to recruit surgeons and institutions with experience in laparoscopic gastrectomy. This was ultimately to evaluate the feasibility of a laparoscopic approach in the forthcoming clinical trials. They first conducted a phase II trial, JCOG0703, with the incidence of anastomotic leakage and pancreatic fistula as the primary end point, enrolled 176 patients, and found the incidence to be 1.7%. [37] Having confirmed the safety of the procedure in this trial, they are currently preparing for a phase III trial with long-term survival as an end point. Again, only early-stage cancers (preoperative diagnosis of T1N0, T1N1, T2 (MP) and T3 (SS) N0) will be eligible. As like mentioned previously, given the small number of events that can be expected from this population, the required sample size to show non-inferiority of the laparoscopic surgery over open surgery (<5% difference in 5-year survival) was calculated to be as much as 920, and the study group expects to complete the recruitment of patients in the following five years. Quality of life assessments using established questionnaires will also be performed among the selected institutions, where sufficient assistance from the clinical research coordinators could be provided.

9. Laparoscopic gastrectomy in the west

In Western countries, a small number of surgeons who challenged this approach did not restrict themselves to T1 stage cancer, [38] because most gastric cancers are diagnosed as locally advanced disease. A small number of studies comparing open and laparoscopic approaches have shown that survival data among those receiving laparoscopy were not inferior to open surgery, although there were significant reductions in pain and incidence of the late postoperative complications. They have not been able to extend their experience to perform a large-scale randomized comparison between laparoscopic and open surgery as they had done with colon cancer, apparently because of the small numbers of operable disease and surgeons who are in capable of performing oncologically safe gastric cancer surgery which is done in East.

The experience in laparoscopic gastrectomy for the treatment of gastric adenocarcinoma in the West has been mostly encouraged in Europe, with a small and limited series of report from the North America and South America published in recent years. In the United States, the first group to describe their experience with laparoscopic gastrectomy with curative intent for GC was Reyes et al. from Mount Sinai Medical Center, in 2001. [39] In this retrospective case-matched study with 36 patients (25 with malignant disease), they compared 18 laparoscopic surgeries with 18 open gastrectomies. Of those with GC, from the laparoscopic group, 9 patients had histologically confirmed adenocarcinoma and 3 with carcinoid tumors compared with 12 adenocarcinomas and 1 gastric lymphoma in the open group. All resected margins in the laparoscopic group were free of tumor, whereas 2 patients in the open group (stages II and III) had R1 resections, likely related to selection bias for these more advanced, open cases. There were no significant differences in extent of lymph node dissection or in intraoperative complications between the two groups. The laparoscopic approach required a significantly longer operative time (4.2 h vs. 3.0 in the open group) likely related to the learning curve of this procedure. However, there were significantly reduced amount of blood loss with fewer transfusions required, earlier return to normal bowel function, lower incidence of the postoperative ileus, and significantly reduced hospital stay in the laparoscopic versus open groups (6.3 vs. 8.6 days).

In 2006, Varela et al. [40] published the second experience with laparoscopic gastrectomy for GC in the United States, representing to date the largest American experience reported. After 15 consecutive laparoscopic gastrectomies, of which 2 were total, 4 proximal, 4 subtotal, 2 distal, and 3 laparoscopic esophagogastrectomies, no conversion to open surgery was reported, and there were no significant differences in operative time, transfusion rate, number of lymph nodes resected, median length of stay, and morbidity, although there was significantly lower blood loss among the laparoscopic group, demonstrating both the feasibility and safety of the laparoscopic approach.

10. Future perspectives

With increasing the experience and the level of the expertise of oncologic surgeons in the minimally invasive approach to gastric resection for cancer, it is becoming evident that laparoscopy, as a surgical modality for gastrectomy, provides equivalent oncologic resections with lymphadenectomy that is comparable to the open approach, with no compromise in terms of the disease recurrence or long-term survival, based on preliminary studies. In addition, based on the known benefits of the minimally invasive approach, including the reduced risks of surgery related trauma, the amount of the blood loss, pain, and earlier recovery for the patient, we are encouraged to expand our indications of laparoscopic surgery. This has been stimulated by the advances in the field of the minimally invasive surgery for benign abdominal disease, and the results from multiple Eastern studies of early-stage cancer. Although an open surgical approach should be applied for any case with concerns of resectibility of the cancer lesion, the safety margin, or capability of operating surgeons , it appears that the minimally invasive surgical approach can be here to stay. However, until more mature long-term follow-up data on advanced gastric cancer treated by minimally invasive approaches are defined, these approaches should be limited to those patients with early- stage gastric cancer. To establish laparoscopic surgery as a standard treatment for advanced gastric cancer, multicenter RCTs comparing the short- and long-term outcomes of laparoscopic surgery versus open surgery are needed. As the indications are continued to expand to treat more advanced tumors and with the supporting data data from the additional prospective studies, we will be able to clearly define the oncologically appropriate application of laparoscopic gastrectomy for all stages of gastric adenocarcinoma.

11. References

[1] Jung KW, Won YJ, Park S, Kong HJ, Sung J, Shin HR, Park EC, Lee JS. Cancer statistics in Korea: incidence, mortality and survival in 2005. J Korean Med Sci. 2009;24:995-1003.

[2] Park CH, Song KY, Kim SN. Treatment results for gastric cancer surgery: 12 years' experience at a single institute in Korea. Eur J Surg Oncol. 2008;34:36-41.

[3] Kitano S, Iso Y, Moriyama M, Sugimachi K. Laparoscopy assisted Billroth I gastrectomy. Surg Laparosc Endosc 1994;4:146–148.

[4] Noshiro H, Nagai E, Shimizu S, et al. Laparoscopically assisted distal gastrectomy with standard radical lymph node dissection for gastric cancer. Surg Endosc 2005;19:1592–1596.

[5] Noh SH, Hyung WJ, Cheong JH. Minimally Invasive Treatment for Gastric Cancer: Approaches and Selection Process. J Surg oncol 2005;90:188-194.

[6] Goh PMY, Tekant Y, Isaac J, et al. The technique of laparoscopic Billroth II gastrectomy. Surg Endosc Laparosc 1992;2: 258–260.

[7] Ohgami M, Otani Y, Kumai K, Kubota T, Kim YI, Kitajima M. Curative laparoscopic surgery for early gastric cancer: 5 years experience. World J Surg 1999;23:187–192.

[8] Ohashi S. Laparoscopic intraluminal (intragastric) surgery for early gastric cancer. A new concept in laparoscopic surgery. Surg Endosc 1995;9:169–171.

[9] Azagra JS, Goergen M, De Simone P, Ibañez-Aguirre J. Minimally invasive surgery for gastric cancer. Surg Endosc 1999;13:351-357.

[10] Kodera Y, Fujiwara M, Ohashi N, Nakayama G, Koike M, Morita S, Nakao A. Laparoscopic surgery for gastric cancer: a collective review with meta-analysis of randomized trials. J Am Coll Surg. 2010;211:677-686.

[11] Lee J, Kim W. Long-term outcomes after laparoscopy-assisted gastrectomy for advanced gastric cancer: analysis of consecutive 106 experiences. J Surg Oncol. 2009;100:693-698.

[12] Lee J, Ryu K, Park S, et al. Learning curve for total gastrectomy with D2 lymph node dissection: cumulative sum analysis for qualified surgery. Ann Surg Oncol 2006;13:1175–1181.

[13] Uyama I, Sugioka A, Fujita J, Komori Y, Matsui H, Hasumi A. Laparoscopic total gastrectomy with distal pancreatosplenectomy and D2 lymphadenectomy for advanced gastric cancer. Gastric Cancer. 1999;2:230-234.

[14] Strong VE, Devaud N, Karpeh M. The role of laparoscopy for gastric surgery in the West. Gastric Cancer. 2009;12:127-131.

[15] Japanese Gastric Cancer Association. Japanese Classification of Gastric Carcinoma; 2nd English Edition. Gastric Cancer 1998;1:10–24.
[16] Cuschieri A, Weeden S, Fielding J, Bancewicz J, Craven J, Joypaul V. Patient survival after D1 and D2 resections for gastric cancer: long-term results of the MRC randomized surgical trial. Surgical Co-operative Group. Br J Cancer 1999;79:1522–1530.
[17] Bonenkamp JJ, Hermans J, Sasako M, van de Velde CJ. Extended lymph-node dissection for gastric cancer. Dutch Gastric Cancer Group. N Engl J Med 1999;340:908–914.
[18] Bunt A, Hermans J, Boon M, van de Velde C, Sasako M, Fleuren G, Bruijin J. Evaluation of the extent of lymphadenectomy in a randomized trial of Western- versus Japanese-type surgery in gastric cancer. J Clin Oncol 1994;12:417–422.
[19] Yasuda K, Shiraishi N, Suematsu T, Yamaguchi K, Adachi Y, Kitano S. Rate of detection of lymph node metastasis is correlated with the depth of submucosal invasion in early stage gastric carcinoma. Cancer 1999;85:2119–2123.
[20] Hyung WJ, Cheong JH, Kim J, Chen J, Choi SH, Noh SH, et al. Application of minimally invasive treatment for early gastric cancer. J Surg Oncol 2004;85:181–185.
[21] Song KY, Kim SN, Park CH. Laparoscopy-assisted distal gastrectomy with D2 lymph node dissection for gastric cancer: technical and oncologic aspects. Surg Endosc 2008;22:655–659.
[22] Tanimura S, Higashino M, Fukunaga Y. et al. Laparoscopic gastrectomy with regional lymph node dissection for upper gastric cancer. Br J Surg 2006;94:204–207.
[23] Park DJ, Lee HJ, Jung HC et al. Clinical outcome of pylorus-preserving gastrectomy in gastric cancer in comparison with conventional distal gastrectomy with Billroth I anastomosis. World J Surg 2008;32:1029–1036.
[24] Shinohara H, Sonoda T, Niki M et al. Laparoscopicallyassisted pylorus-preserving gastrectomy with preservation of the vagus nerve. Eur J Surg 2002168:55–58.
[25] Sano T, Hollowood A. Early gastric cancer: diagnosis and less invasive treatments. Scand J Surg. 2006;95:249-255.
[26] Kitano S, Shiraishi N, Fujii K, et al. A randomized controlled trial comparing open vs laparoscopy-assisted distal gastrectomy for the treatment of early gastric cancer: An interim report. Surgery 2002;131(1 Suppl):S306-311.
[27] Huscher CGS, Mingoli A, Sgarzini G, Sansonetti A, Paola MD, Recher A, et al. Laparoscopic versus open subtotal gastrectomy for distal gastric cancer: five-year results of a randomized prospective trial. Ann Surg 2005;241:232–237.
[28] Kim H, Hyung W, Cho G, et al. Morbidity and mortality of laparoscopic gastrectomy versus open gastrectomy for gastric cancer: an interim report—a phase III multicenter, prospective, randomized trial (KLASS Trial). Ann Surg 2010;251:417–420.
[29] Kodera Y, Fujiwara M, Ohashi N, Nakayama G, Koike M, Morita S, Nakao A. Laparoscopic surgery for gastric cancer: a collective review with meta-analysis of randomized trials. J Am Coll Surg. 2010;211:677-686.
[30] Lee J, Han H. A prospective randomized study comparing open vs laparoscopy-assisted distal gastrectomy in early gastric cancer:early results. Surg Endosc 2005;19:168–173.

[31] Fujiwara M, Kodera Y, Misawa K, et al. Longterm outcomes of early-stage gastric carcinoma patients treated with laparoscopyassisted surgery. J Am Coll Surg 2008;206:138–143.
[32] Lee SW, Nomura E, Bouras G, Tokuhara T, Tsunemi S, Tanigawa N. Long-term oncologic outcomes from laparoscopic gastrectomy for gastric cancer: a single-center experience of 601 consecutive resections. J Am Coll Surg. 2010;211:33-40.
[33] Kitano S, Shiraishi N, Uyama I, et al. A multicenter study on oncologic outcome of laparoscopic gastrectomy for early cancer in Japan. Ann Surg 2007;245:68–72.
[34] Song J, Lee H, Cho G, et al. Recurrence following laparoscopy assisted gastrectomy for gastric cancer: a multicenter retrospective analysis of 1,417 patients. Ann Surg Oncol 2010;17:1777–1786.
[35] Huscher CG, Mingoli A, Sgarzini G, Sansonetti A, Di Paola M, Recher A, Ponzano C. Laparoscopic versus open subtotal gastrectomy for distal gastric cancer: five-year results of a randomized prospective trial. Ann Surg. 2005;241:232-237.
[36] Kim W, Song KY, Lee HJ, Han SU, Hyung WJ, Cho GS. The impact of comorbidity on surgical outcomes in laparoscopy-assisted distal gastrectomy: a retrospective analysis of multicenter results. Ann Surg. 2008;248:793-799.
[37] Katai H, Sasako M, Fukuda H, Nakamura K, Hiki N, Saka M, Yamaue H, Yoshikawa T, Kojima K; JCOG Gastric Cancer Surgical Study Group. Safety and feasibility of laparoscopy-assisted distal gastrectomy with suprapancreatic nodal dissection for clinical stage I gastric cancer: a multicenter phase II trial (JCOG 0703). Gastric Cancer. 2010;13:238-244.
[38] Strong V, Devaud N, Allen P, et al. Laparoscopic versus open subtotal gastrectomy for adenocarcinoma: a case-control study. Ann Surg Oncol 2009;16:1507–1513.
[39] Reyes CD, Weber KJ, Gagner M, Divino CM. Laparoscopic vs open gastrectomy. A retrospective review. Surg Endosc 2001;15:928–931.
[40] Varela JE, Hiyashi M, Nguyen T, Sabio A, Wilson SE, Nguyen NT. Comparison of laparoscopic and open gastrectomy for gastric cancer. Am J Surg 2006;192:837–842.

6

Lymph Node Dissection

Bulent Cavit Yuksel, Okan Murat Akturk and Ilyas Hakan Ozel
Ankara Numune Training and Research Hospital
Turkey

1. Introduction

Gastric cancer remains as one of the leading causes of death worldwide (Yoshida et al., 2004). Middle third and distal cancers tend to decline worldwide. However, in the western populations proximal gastric cancers tend to increase even though the incidence of those cancers stays the same in Japan. Today, the incidence of early gastric cancer has reached above 50% in Japan while in the west two thirds of gastric cancers are at an advanced stage at the time of diagnosis (Biondi, 2010). This problem is complicated further by a recurrence rate of 40% to 65% in patients resected with curative intent (Dicken, 2005). Currently, the only potentially curative option for gastric cancer is surgery which may promise complete resection, although the extent of regional lymphadenectomy (LND) has been a matter of considerable debate.

2. Surgery of the stomach

Radical resection of stomach and the related lymphatic drainage has been the way of treatment of gastric cancer (GC) in west and Japan. The debate has been carried out on what extent the resection must be carried out. Japanese investigators assert that the extended LND (D2) removes tumor in the regional lymph nodes (LNs) before it can metastasize. In addition, it is argued that extended LND improves staging accuracy. On the other hand, western surgeons have argued that the benefits promised by extended lymphadenectomy may be reversed by the high complication rate even if they have any. Theoretically, the removal of a wider range of LNs by extended LN dissection increases the chances for cure. In fact, the pattern of recurrence after extended surgery is completely different from that after limited surgery and involves locoregional recurrence in the majority of cases (Gunderson & Sosin, 1982). An extended LN dissection might have an influence on the locoregional recurrence rate. However, if the patients have already developed micrometastases or if no LNs are affected, such resection might be irrelevant and harmful, in terms of increased morbidity and mortality (Tanizawa & Terashima, 2010).

2.1 The classification of lymph node tiers

The Japanese Research Society for the study of gastric cancer published a manual in 1963 standardizing LND and pathologic evaluations for GC; these guidelines recognized 16 different LN stations that surround the stomach. These 16 nodal stations are grouped according to the location and extension of the primary tumor (N0-N4) and the extent of lymphadenectomy is classified according the level of LND (D1-D4). In D1 dissections, only the perigastric nodes directly attached along the lesser curvature and greater curvatures of the stomach are removed (stations 1-6, N1 level). An incomplete N1 dissection is labelled a D0 lymphadenectomy. D2 dissections (N2 level) add the removal of nodes along the left gastric artery (station 7), common hepatic artery (station 8), celiac trunk (station 9), splenic hilus, and splenic artery (station 10 and 11). D3 dissections include the dissection of lymph nodes at stations 12 through 14, along the hepatoduodenal ligament and the root of the mesentery (N3 level). Finally D4 resections add the stations 15 and 16 in the paraaortic and the paracolic region (N4 level). The incidence of metastasis to any perigastric station is highest when the tumor location is close to it. There is little variation in the metastatic pattern along the lesser curvature between tumors of different thirds. For tumors of antrum right paracadiac lymph nodes are staged as second tier while left paracardiac lymph nodes are N3. For tumors of cardia the 5th and 6th lymph node stations are in the second tier (Kim et al., 2001) .

2.2 The regional lymph nodes

No. 1 Right paracardial LN
No. 2 Left paracardial LN
No. 3 LN along the lesser curvature
No. 4sa LN along the short gastric vessels
No. 4sb LN along the left gastroepiploic vessels
No. 4d LN along the right gastroepiploic vessels
No. 5 Suprapyloric LN
No. 6 Infrapyloric LN
No. 7 LN along the left gastric artery
No. 8a LN along the common hepatic artery (Anterosuperior group)
No. 8p LN along the common hepatic artery (Posterior group)
No. 9 LN around the celiac artery
No. 10 LN at the splenic hilum
No. 11p LN along the proximal splenic artery
No. 11d LN along the distal splenic artery
No. 12a LN in the hepatoduodenal ligament (along the hepatic artery)
No. 12b LN in the hepatoduodenal ligament (along the bile duct)
No. 12p LN in the hepatoduodenal ligament (behind the portal vein)
No. 13 LN on the posterior surface of the pancreatic head
No. 14v LN along the superior mesenteric vein
No. 14a LN along the superior mesenteric artery
No. 15 LN along the middle colic vessels
No. 16a1 LN in the aortic hiatus
No. 16a2 LN around the abdominal aorta (from the upper margin of the celiac trunk to the lower margin of the left renal vein)
No. 16b1 LN around the abdominal aorta (from the lower margin of the left renal vein to the upper margin of the inferior mesenteric artery)
No. 16b2 LN around the abdominal aorta (from the upper margin of the inferior mesenteric artery to the aortic bifurcation)
No. 17 LN on the anterior surface of the pancreatic head

No. 18 LN along the inferior margin of the pancreas
No. 19 Infradiaphragmatic LN
No. 20 LN in the esophageal hiatus of the diaphragm
No. 110 Paraesophageal LN in the lower thorax
No. 111 Supradiaphragmatic LN
No. 112 Posterior mediastinal LN

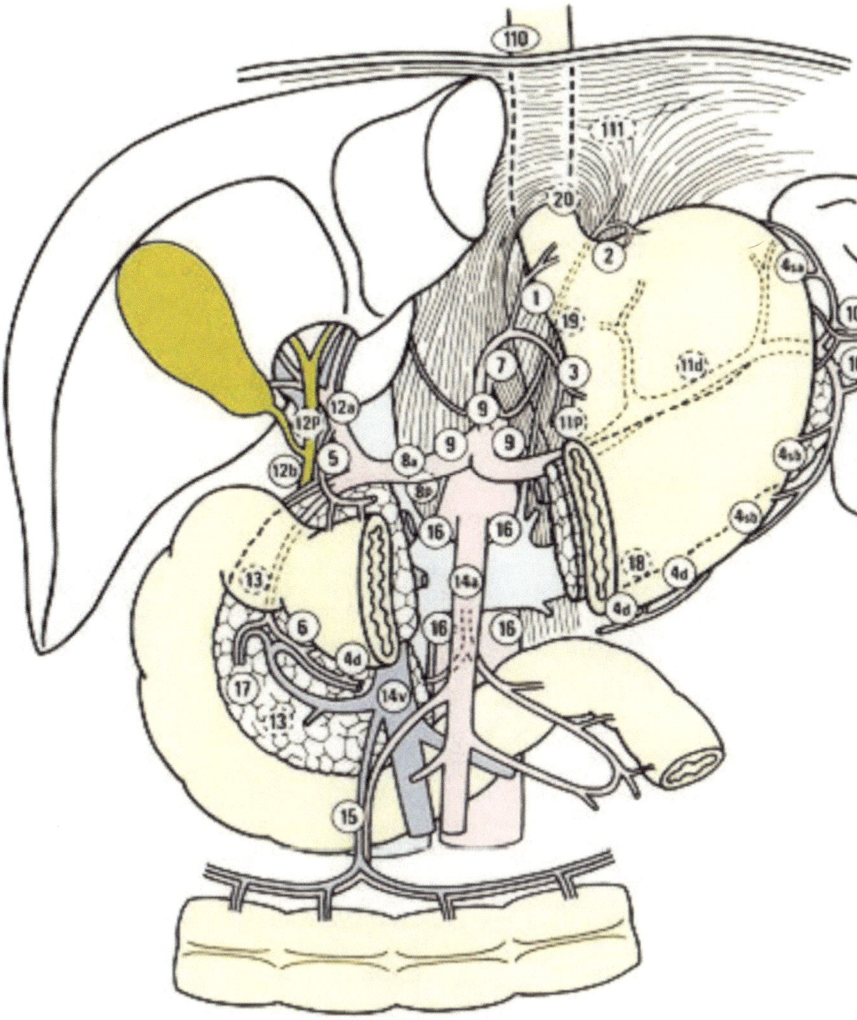

Fig. 1. The lymph node stations according to the Japanese classification

R0 resection indicates a microscopically margin-negative resection, in which no gross or microscopic tumor remains in the primary tumor bed. R1 resection indicates the removal of all macroscopic disease but microscopic margins are positive for tumors. R2 indicates gross residual disease with gross residual tumor that was not resected (primary tumor, regional nodes and macroscopic margin involvement). Resection in the eastern world is a little more

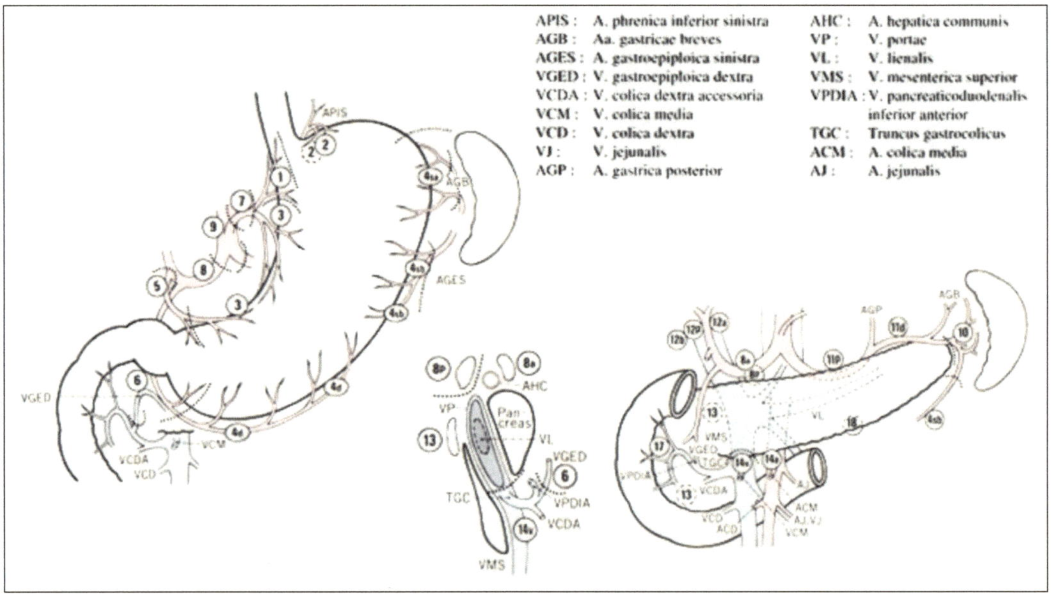

Fig. 2. Location of lymph nodes around abdominal aorta.

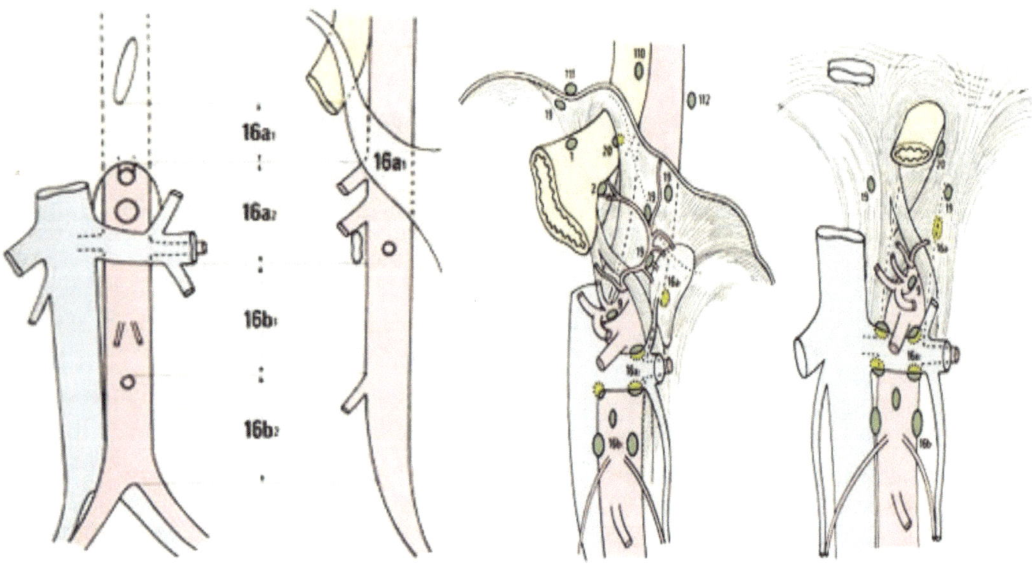

Fig. 3. Location of lymph nodes in the esophageal hiatus, and infradiaphragmatic and paraaortic regions.

complicated: Resection A: no residual disease, with a high cure probability. It implies resections satisfying all of the following conditions: tumor without serosal invasion; N0 treated by D1, D2, or D3 lymph node dissections, or tumor with first-level lymph node treated by D2 or D3 resection; no distant, peritoneal or liver metastases, negative cytological examination of peritoneal fluid and proximal and distal margins > 10 mm. Resection B: no histopathologic residual disease but not fulfilling criteria for resection A. Resection C: definite residual disease (Biondi, 2010).

The groups of lymph node stations used to define the extent of lymph node dissection

	Location of the tumor			
Station Number	A, AM	M, MA, MC	C,CM	AMC,MAC, MCA,CMA
1	N2	N1	N1	N1
2	N3	N2	N1	N1
3,4	N1	N1	N1	N1
5,6	N1	N1	N2	N1
7,8,9	N2	N2	N2	N2
10,11	N3	N2	N2	N2
12,13,14	N3	N3	N3	N3
15,16	N4	N4	N4	N4

A: Antrum, M: Middle, C: Cardia

Table 1. Groups of lymph node stations used to define the extent of lymph node dissection.

The Union Internationale Contrale Cancer (UICC)/American Joint Committee on Cancer (AJCC) classification, which is most widely used for the staging of gastric cancer, suggests that at least 15 lymph nodes should be examined for a correct assessment of N staging. Lymph node dissemination is in an orderly fashion through lymphatic channels in gastric cancer (Shi & Zou, 2010). However, the type of fixative and clearance solution used by a pathology department may influence the number of nodes examined. One study found that 78% of nodes <5 mm are missed by the routine formalin fixation that is used in most Western countries, whereas clearance solutions allow detection of nodes 1 mm in diameter (Herrera & Villareal, 1992). Studies estimate that LNs will be involved with tumors for 3–5% of cases of gastric adenocarcinoma limited to the mucosa; 11–25% of cases for those limited to the sub-mucosa; 50% for T2; and 83% for T3 tumors (Coburn, 2009).
The 7th editon has brought some changes.
N0 (N plus zero): The cancer has not spread into the regional lymph nodes.
N1: The cancer has spread to one to two regional lymph nodes.
N2: The cancer has spread to three to six regional lymph nodes.
N3: The cancer has spread to seven or more regional lymph nodes.
N3a: The cancer has spread to seven to 15 regional lymph nodes.
N3b: The cancer has spread to more than 16 regional lymph nodes.
As a critics to TNM classification, it is difficult to directly correlate the number of lymph nodes assessed with the extent of lymphadenectomy. Autopsy studies have shown that an average of 15 nodes can be harvested from a D1 lymphadenectomy, 27 nodes from a D2 lymphadenectomy, and 43 nodes from a D3 lymphadenectomy (Wagner et al., 1991). But studies have shown the TNM classification to be an easier way with a more accurate prognostic value. But since the fifth edition prior to 1997 AJCG system was based on anatomic location of involved nodes rather than their number. Positive nodes >3 cm from the primary tumor or nodes associated with celiac or celiac based arteries were deemed N2 nodes. However, this anatomic scheme caused some problems undermining the concept of

anatomical staging. For example, following surgical resection some surgeon-pathologist teams harvested nodes on fresh specimens whereas others would harvest nodes only after fixation and substantial contraction of the specimen, the alterations that resulted from these different techniques compromised the staging accuracy. Besides, many surgeons in the west excluded the N2 node dissection and that also impaired the quality of accurate staging when a higher number of lymph nodes were extracted from a D2 resection. Thus, interpretation was harder as Japanese and German surgeons perfomed mainly D2 resection while at that time many surgeons in other countries in west ignored D2 resection and thus stage migration effect again vitiated the accurate staging. Therefore, in the western world the TNM clasisification has gained wider ground because of better prognostic predictions it has offered as justified by Japanese surgeons.

A number of investigators have observed progressive decrease in survival with the increasing number of involved lymph nodes, with an appearent drop off in survival when 3 or more nodes are involved. Another drop off have been reported when more than 6 nodes are involved. Involvement beyond 15 or 16 nodes has been observed to be largely incompetent with long term survival(Hundahl, 2002). As a prognostic tool, ratio between metastatic lymph nodes and the total number of lymph nodes examined was proposed(Marchet, 2007). Several cutoff were studied increasing in pentathonic or decimal scale starting from zero to mostly >30 %; the survival decreases as the involved lymph node ratio increases. In a study by Xu et al. it is proposed that this scheme may also be usefull for patients who had lower than 15 lymph nodes dissected (Xu et al.,2009) .

2.2 Patterns of relapse and metastasis

In striving to achieve cure for gastric cancer it is essential to understand the modes of spread and patterns of relapse. Only then an optimum treatment with reasonable expectations are possible. The metastatic pathways are:

2.2.1 Direct extension

Into neighbouring organs and structures generally resected en-bloc with the stomach. Once a lesion has extended beyond the gastric wall, a multitude of organs and structures can be involved, dependent on lesion location within the stomach. For proximal lesions, organs or structures that may be involved with superior or anterior extragastric extension include the left diaphragm, anterior abdominal wall, or undersurface of the liver, while with posterior extension, the celiac artery, body of pancreas (anterior, superior), aorta, or diaphragmatic crura may be involved. For body of stomach lesions, anterior extension may involve the anterior abdominal wall or liver; lateral extension--the gastrosplenic ligament or spleen; posterior extension—the pancreas (tail, body); superior extension—the gastrohepatic ligament or lesser omentum; and inferior extension--the transverse colon or mesocolon, or greater omentum. With distal gastric lesions, posterior extension may involve the head of pancreas or porta hepatis structures; inferior extension--the transverse mesocolon and colon. Adherence from inflammatory conditions can mimic direct extension of tumor, but all adhesions between a gastric carcinoma and adjacent structures must be regarded as malignant (Gunderson, 2002).

2.2.2 Lymphatic route

Lymphatic spread occurs via subserosal and submucosal lymphatic plexuses depending on the depth of invasion. The lymphatic drainage of the stomach follows the arterial supply.

Although most lymphatics ultimately drain into the celiac nodal area, lymph drainage sites can include the splenic hilum, suprapancreatic nodal groups, porta hepatis, and gastroduodenal areas. Abundant lymphatic channels are present within both the submucosal and subserosal layers of the gastric wall. Microscopic or subclinical spread well beyond the visible gross lesion occurs via these lymphatic channels (intramural spread), and the surgeon can be misled into thinking that resection margins are free of tumor. Accordingly, frozen sections of the gastric resection margins should be obtained intraoperatively to ensure that margins of resection are microscopically uninvolved. The submucosal lymphatic plexus is also prominent in the esophagus and the subserosal plexus in the duodenum, allowing both proximal and distal intramural tumor spread. Although a so-called "duodenal block" occurs with the mucosa scarcely ever being involved for more than 1-2 mm beyond the pylorus, the existence of a prominent subserosal plexus allows distal spread in as high as 30% to 40% of patients (Gunderson, 2002). In the stomach, as in other organs, the very presence of cancer can alter the normal lymphatic drainage. Obstructed vessels can divert the drainage so that metastases appear in unexpected nodes. Collateral lymphatics can form, producing a shift in the drainage pattern. The possibly multicentric origin of gastric cancer further complicates a simple approach to the proposed resection (Fischer & Bland, 2007).

2.2.3 Peritoneal disease

Because stomach is a peritoneal organ once the tumor cells have extended beyond the gastric wall to the serosal surface peritoneal spread may happen. Peritoneal spread may initially be a localized process confined to the surrounding ligaments (Gunderson, 1982) .

2.2.4 Hematogenous spread

For malignancies confined to the stomach the venous drainage is primarily to liver which proves an effective filter. As neoplastic cells invade beyond the stomach wall into adjacent organs, hematogeanous spread through the lymphatics and venous system of the involved organ happens and metastasis to lungs and other organs may happen (Smalley et al., 2002).

2.3 Patterns of relapse

There are 5 ways recurrence following surgical removal of gastric carcinoma: lymph node, remnant stomach, local, peritoneal and hematogenous recurrence. Sixty percent to 72% of gastric cancer patients succumb to recurrences within the first 2 Hematogenous or lymphatic spreads without intraabdominal metastases occur rarely. It may be postulated that gastric cancer prefers to spread intraabdominally, and that locoregional control is therefore an important issue in treatment strategy years (Wu, 2003).. Locoregional recurrence rates varies from 25% to 96% depending on different detection methods and study populations.

2.4 Histology and recurrence

Gastric cancer can recur in different pathways. The possibility of predicting the risk and type of recurrence in patients with resectable gatric cancer could have important implications for therapy, both in the surgical aproach (extent of lymphadenectomy, partial or total resection) and in complemetary therapies. Marelli et al. found out that the main difference was found on the onset of peritoneal recurrence in a study of 412 patients in which they compared the recurrence patterns of intestinal type and diffuse type years (Marelli et al., 2002). Shiriashi et al. confirmed that most recurrences were within the first two years after surgery and rare after 5 years (Shiriashi et al., 2000).

For intestinal type of the tumor lymph node positivity, depth of invasion, advanced age and male gender significantly increases the risk of recurrence. The patterns of relapse were mainly locoregional or hematogenous and peritoneal recurrence was limited. For diffuse type of tumors very high rates of peritoneal recurrence were observed in neoplasms with infiltration of the serosa, involvement of second level lymph nodes, and large tumor size. Locoregional recurrences were frequent in advanced forms, lymph node–positive cases, and tumors larger than 4 cm. The rate of hematogenous recurrence was generally smaller than that of peritoneal or locoregional disease. Early forms and tumors smaller than 4 cm recurred primarily via hematogenous route.

The main difference was found in the onset of peritoneal recurrence; this was observed in 34% of diffuse-type cases compared to 9% of intestinal-type cases, and was the main pathway of spread in the former. Compared to intestinal-type cells, the diffuse type showed a greater predisposition to proliferate in the peritoneum, considering that 50% of the cases with infiltration of the serosa led to peritoneal carcinomatosis, which was observed in only 16% of T3 and T4 intestinal-type cases. On the contrary, recurrences of intestinal-type tumors were mainly locoregional or hematogenous. The incidence of hematogenous recurrence did not show significant differences between the intestinal and the diffuse types; in both groups of patients, they observed a higher frequency of this recurrence in lymph node–positive cases, a finding in accord with other reports. However, the degree of involvement in the various organs was different, because the intestinal type metastasized primarily to the liver, whereas in the diffuse type the liver was involved in only half of the cases; in the other cases, hematogenous metastases involved distant organs. The data may suggest that in the diffuse type, but not in the intestinal type, superextended lymphadenectomy may play a more important role in reducing the risk of recurrence. The diffuse type may show a greater propensity than the intestinal type to metastasize to third- and fourth-level lymph nodes (Marelli et al., 2002).

In a large series Nakamura et al. demonstrated that there is some correlation between the tumor histological type and the gross type. Seventy nine percent of diffusely infiltrating tumors and 69% of ulcerative infiltrating tumors were poorly differentiated and 60% of polipoid tumors were well differentiated in advanced carcinomas. In early carcinomas 89% of Type 1 and 77% of Type IIa lesions were well differentiated. Type llc tumors were either well (31%), moderate(19%) or poorly differentiated (50%). In their large series of 10 thousand patients the most frequently encountered macroscopic type of advanced cacinoma was the ulcerative infiltrating tumor (41%), followed by ulcerating circumscribed type(31%). In early carcinomas type llc (70%) was the most frequently encountered type, followed by Type II a. In advanced forms well differentiated types showed fairer prognosis (Nakamura et al., 1992).

Adachi et al. demonstrated that patients with poorly differentiated type show a poorer prognosis especially when the tumor is bigger than 10 cm or serosal involvement is positive. If the tumor did not invade serosa but had lymph node metastasis, survival rate was signifcantly lower in the well differentiated group. Moriguchi et al. also demostrated that when the tumor invasion was restricted within mucosa or submucosa the well differentiated type of tumor were associated with poorer pognosis. This difference can be explained by the characteristics of well differentiated type which readily develops blood-bourne metastases irrespective of the degree of penetration by tumor cells (Adachi et al.,1997).

2.5 Lymph nodes and tumors of cardia

Tumors of cardia are generally larger than the tumors of other parts of the stomach. The incidence of serosal invasion, lymph node metastasis and lymphatic and blood vessel invasion are higher. With regards to the site of recurrence both lymph node and hematogenous recurrence were observed more frequently in the cardia than remaining parts of the stomach. The adenocarcinoma of gastric cardia shows involvement of left and right paracardial section and the lesser curvature as the predominating areas, then the lower posterior mediastinum and left gastric artery and abdominal aorta(Saito et al., 2006). The incidence of lymph nodes at the splenic hilum and splenic artery are less, between 9% and 20%. The splenic hilar lymph node metastasis increases with the advanced stage(Shin et al., 2009). In a review of literature by Ashikaga et al. the incidence of hilar lymph node positivity for T1 tumors of cardia is 0,3%, for subserosal involvement the incidence is %13 and 26% when the tumor has infiltrated serosa. The involvement of the hilar lymph node is associated with ominous prognosis (Shin et al., 2009).

For tumors of cardia in order to decide the necessity of dissection No 10 lymph nodes, evaluation of the 4d lymph node metastasis has been proposed. If the 4d lymph nodes are uninvolved it is unlikely for the splenic hilus lymph nodes to be involved (Ishikawa et al., 2009).

2.6 Lymphadenectomy and pancreaticosplenectomy

Tumors of the upper and middle stomach are known to metastasize to the splenic artery (station 11) and splenic hilar (station 10) lymph nodes, and distal pancreatectomy and splenectomy were historically routinely performed to clear these nodal stations. Pancreatic fistula rates were high, thus significantly increasing the morbidity of the D2 lymphadenectomy procedure (Yoon et al., 2009). Maruyama et al. described a pancreas-preserving D2 lymphadenectomy that resected the spleen and splenic artery along with the station 10 and 11 lymph nodes(Maruyama et al., 1995). A retrospective study from Japan of nearly 400 patients found that there was no survival benefit in patients undergoing total gastrectomy combined with distal pancreatectomy and splenectomy over patients undergoing total gastrectomy with splenectomy only (Kitamura et al., 1999). Distal pancreatectomy is now generally considered to be unwarranted in the routine performance of a D2 lymphadenectomy until there is direct extension of the tumor. A retrospective Japanese study of 224 patients with proximal gastric cancer found no survival benefit in patients who received pancreaticosplenectomy or splenectomy over pancreas and spleen preservation, but morbidity was significantly greater in the pancreaticosplenectomy group (Kodera et al., 1997). Sasako et al. estimated the benefit of dissecting the station 10 and 11 lymph nodes for a proximal gastric cancer at 5.6% (Sasako et al., 1995). Hartgrink et al. analyzed the patients in the Dutch Gastric Cancer Trial who had lymph node metastases at stations 10 and 11. Of the 18 patients with station 10 metastases, the 11-year survival rate was 11%. Of the 24 patients with station 11 metastases, the 11-year survival rate was 8%. The authors concluded that "the relevance of the dissection of these nodes has to be questioned as the survival benefit is small and morbidity and hospital mortality are significantly increased" (Hartgrink et al., 2005).

Although most expert gastric cancer surgeons no longer resect the distal pancreas as part of a D2 lymphadenectomy unless there is direct tumor extension, the resection of the spleen continues to be controversial (Yoon et al., 2009). Two prospective randomized trials of total gastrectomy and lymphadenectomy with or without splenectomy have been performed in Chile and South Korea. Both studies found no difference in overall survival, and the Chilean study found a significantly higher rate of infectious complications in the splenectomy group. However, the number of patients in these studies was between 187–207, and thus the power of these studies to determine a modest improvement in survival for splenectomy is limited(Csendes et al., 2002, Yu et al., 2006).

3. Scientific basis of lymph node dissection

3.1 The Japanese evidence

In the western world the over-all 5-year survival rate among patients with resectable gastric cancers range from 10%-30%, while in Japan the survival for the same subgroup of patients is between 50% and 62% largely attributable to the lymph node dissection known as D2 which was introduced in 1960s. In Japan standard resection refers to total or subtotal gastrectomy with D2 resection. The 5 year survival rate following D2 lymphadenectomy is 63,8% and is superior to survival after D1 or D0 lymphadenecomy (41,2% and 20,3% respectively) according to the Japanese Nationwide Registry for Gastric Cancer. The major effect of systemic lymph node dissection is the reduction in locoregional recurrence. The proportions of local recurrences were decreased by the introduction of this procedure, 38% in 1967-1971, 12% in 1982-1986. Operative mortality rate is very low in Japanese series and no different from D1/D0 patients. According to the Japanese Natiowide registry reports the 30 days postoperative mortality is 1,7% (Maruyama et al., 1998).

3.2 The evidence for D2 resection in western world

The National Comprehensive Cancer Network (NCCN), an alliance of 21 of the world's leading cancer center has released a latest guideline in 2010. According to this guideline gastric resection should include the regional lymphatics, the perigastric lymph nodes as well as those along the celiac axis with at least 15 lymph nodes. Splenectomy is acceptable only when spleen or hilus is involved. The guideline points out several studies the guideline is based on.

Schwarz et al. reviewed relationships between the number of LNs examined and survival among the patients in SEER (Surveillance, Epidemiology and End Results) database. Outcomes were analyzed only for the stage subgroups characterized by the N categories N2 or N3, and transmural tumor extension (T categories T2b or T3). Advanced but potentially still curable gastric cancer (stages IIIA, IIIB, or stage IV M0) is associated with very high recurrence rates after gastrectomy. For every ten extra LNs added to the total LN count, the calculated overall survival increased by: 5.7% (T2b-3N2), 4.6% (T2b-3N3), or 5.9%. Despite the small incremental increases in survival, benefits based on increasing LN counts were obvious for all groups analyzed, but reached statistically significant differences only for the N3 subgroup. The findings demonstrate that even in transmural or serosa-positive gastric cancer with advanced nodal involvement, more extensive LN dissection and analysis influences survival. Stage-based survival prediction of advanced gastric cancer without distant metastases depends on total LN number and number of negative LNs. For the curative-intent gastrectomy of locoregionally advanced gastric cancer, retrieval and examination of larger numbers of LNs are suggested. It is criticized that recommended minimum goal of 15 LNs to satisfy current (6th edition at the time the study was made) AJCC staging criteria appears insufficient . Especially for N3 categories, the minimum goal theoretically should be set to at least ten LNs above the number of positive nodes. Practically, this would require at least 25 LNs although counts of 40 or more total LNs appear even yet superior. As long as operative morbidity is not affected negatively, extended lymphadecectomy (ELND) during potentially curative gastrectomy is recommended even for advanced gastric cancer. The NCNN guideline excerpts that patients who had more than 15 D2 lymph nodes and patients with more than 20 N3 lymph nodes dissected had the best survival outcome (Schwarz & Smith, 2007). As a result the NCNN guide has increased the number of lyph nodes necessarily dissected for better staging and curativeness in the seventh edition. There is now a cathegory of N3b with metastases to 16 or more lymph nodes.

3.2.1 The Dutch study from the beginning to now

The Dutch gastric cancer group randomized 711 patients to go under resection with curative intent, and randomly assigned them into D1 (380 patients) and D2 (311patients) resection groups. The results of this study is extensively eveluated. They demostrated that patients in D2 goup suffered from a higher rate of postoperative complications than did those in D1 group (43% vs 25%), higher postoperative mortality rates (10% vs 4%) and longer hospital stay (Bonenkamp et al., 1995). Nevertheless, they found out that the 5-year survival rate did not significantly differ between the two groups; 45% in D1 group and 47% in D2 group (Bonenkamp et al., 1999). After a median follow up period of 11 years no statistically survival difference was encountered between the two groups (D1 30% vs D2 35%) (Hartgrink,2004). Noncompliance, which is inadequate removal of 2nd echelon and contamination, which is unnecessary removal of the second tier lymph nodes were encountered. In Dutch trial while 6% of the patients who were supposedly to go under D1 resection had additional lymph node dissections, 51% of the patients with D2 resection had one or more node stations left undissected (Bonenkamp et al., 1998).

The learning curve for D2 resection is steep and it has been proposed that it may entail as much as 25 operations. The higher complication rates maybe attributed to the lack of experience of the participating surgeons with D2 resection but in subgroup analysis higher morbdity and mortality rates are asscoiated with pancreaticosplenectomy carried out in the D2 group, which was regarded as a part of the R0 surgery especially for proximal cancers at the time of the study (de Gara et al., 2003).

The Dutch gastric study revealed a 30% stage migration when a higher number of lymph nodes were examined. The most prominent feature is that patients with N2 disease in the D2 group showed significantly improved survival rates than those in D1 group (%19 vs 0%) in consistence with that in the subgroup analysis Siewart et al. had demonstrated a significant difference in patients with stages ll and llla in the German study. In the long term follow up the results of the Dutch study confers a lower risk of recurrence in patients who underwent D2 resection and higher survival rates.

In the final analysis of 15 years follow up which was evauated in a 2010 article gastric-cancer-related death rate was significantly higher in the D2 group (48%, 182 patients) compared with the D1 group (37%, 123 patients), whereas death due to other diseases was similar in both groups. Local recurrence was 22% (82 patients) in the D1 group versus 12%

(40 patients) in D2, and regional recurrence was 19% (73 patients) in D1 versus 13% (43 patients) in D2.

Even though the initial conclusions from the Dutch gastric cancer study were discouraging especially when a high mortality rate was observed without any significant survival improvement, on the final conclusion D2 lymphadenectomy is the recommended surgical approach for patients with resectable (curable) gastric cancer while especially a spleen preserving technique is available (Songun et al., 2010).

3.2.2 The German study

A total of 1654 patients treated for gastric cancer between 1986 and 1989 at 19 centers in Germany and Austria were included. The resected specimen were evaluated histopathologically according to a standardized protocol. The extent of lymphadenectomy was classified after surgery based on the number of removed lymph nodes on histopathologic assessment (25 or fewer removed nodes, Dl or standard lymphadenectomy; >25 removed nodes, D2 or extended lymphadenectomy). Endpoint of the study was death. Median follow-up of the surviving patients was 8.4 years. There was no difference in the postsurgical morbidity and mortality rates between patients with standard and extended lymph node dissection, even though they were worse when compared to Japanese statistics. The 30- and 90-day mortality rates in the total patient population were 5.1% and 10.6%, respectively.

Calculated 10-year survival rate was 26.3% ± 4.7% in the total patient population and 36.1% ± 1.6% in those with an R0 resection. Extended lymph node dissection significantly increased the 10-year survival rate and median survival time in patients with UICC stage II tumors. In this patient subgroup, extended lymphadenectomy resulted in a marked improvement of the 10-year survival rate from 19.9% with standard lymphadenectomy to 49.2% with extended lymphadenectomy (Siewart et al., 1998).

3.2.3 The British study

In 1986 the Medical Research Council of Great Britain iniated a nationwide, multicenter randomized controlled trial (RCT) comparing D1 dissection to D2 dissection of 200 patients randomized at each limb. Postoperative mortality was significantly higher in the D2 group than D1 (13,1% vs 6,5%). postoperative complications were also higher in the D2 group reaching 46%. However, in this trial many surgeons thought that D2 dissection included splenectomy and splenectomy was carried out in many distal gastrectomy cases (Cushieri et al., 1999) Pancreaticosplenectomy was carried out in 56% of the cases in D2 group. Splenectomy with subtotal gastrectomy causes serious ischemia of the remnant stomach causing anastomotic leakage or necrosis. The five year overall survival did not differ in either limb (Tanizawa & Terashima, 2010).

3.2.4 Italian study

The majority of complications in the Dutch and British trials are associated with pancreticosplenectomy. Deguili et al. have shown the safety of D2 dissection with pancreas preservation. In their studies postoperative morbidity is as low as 13-17% with mortality rates 0,6-3% without significant difference in mortality and morbidity between D1 and D2 results. In their IGCSG-R01 trial splenopancreatectomy was not considered as a routine part of the D2 total gastrectomy. The spleen was removed according to the Maruyama technique only when the tumour was in the left part of the upper stomach or located close to the greater curvature, beyond Demel's point. The spleen was also preserved in patients with clinical T1 tumours. The pancreas was removed only when tumour involvement was suspected. As a consequence the overall morbidity rate after D2 and D1 dissections was 17.9% and 12.0%. The postoperative 30-day mortality rate was 3.0%after D1 and 2.2% after D2 gastrectomy. In specialized centres the rate of complications following D2 dissection is much lower than in published randomized Western trials. D2 dissection, in an appropriate setting, can therefore be considered a safe option for the radical management of gastric cancer in Western patients (Deguili et al., 2004).

3.2.5 Additional information

Diaz et al. studied prospectively 126 consecutive patients operated upon for gastric cancer, with gastrectomy and D2 lymphadenectomy. Hospital morbidity and mortality, relapses, and patient survival after 5 years were studied. The overall hospital mortality rate was 1.6%, with a mortality of 2.1% in the patients submitted to total gastrectomy. The overall morbidity rate was 29.4% with a 5-year survival of more than 50%. Dehiscence of the esophagojejunal anastomosis was recorded in 1.6%. The median follow-up was 73.6 months. Relapses were observed in 37% of the patients (76% in the fi rst 2 years). Overall actuarial survival after 5 years was 52.3%, and 5-year survival in the patients with R0 resection with positive N2 lymph nodes according to the Japanese classification was 26.5% (Diaz et al., 2008).

Other reports from Spain reveal results comparable to Japanese practice applying the D2 resection. Sierra et al.(2003) found no significant difference in the length of hospital stay (median, 12.1 and 13.1 days), overall morbidity (48.2% and 53.5%), or operative mortality (2.3% and 0%) between D1 and D2, respectively. Five-year survival in the D2 group was longer (50.6%) than in the D1 group (41.4%) for tumor stages (tumor-node-metastasis) greater than l .

An RCT performed in the USA investigated the role of post-operative chemoradiotherapy and also showed significant survival benefit . However, only 10% of the patients underwent D2 dissection, there was a very high rate of local recurrence, and the surgery was not standardized among the participating hospitals. Subgroup analysis found survival benefit only in D0 or D1, but not in the D2-dissected group(Mac Donald et al., 2001). The study thus showed that D0/D1 dissection was insufficient treatment .

There are reports about low mortality and morbidity for D2 dissection from various european countries. For example, the Latvian Oncology Center in a series of 468 patients has in hospital mortality 3,3% and morbidity 16,3% with a five year overall survival of 52,5%. The 5 year survival rates according to pT cathegory are 86% for pT1, 65% for pT2 and 43% for pT3, 27% for pT4 (Sivins et al., 2009).

3.3 D2 vs D3

In a review by Tanizawa and Terashima three major studies comparing D2 lymphadectomy with D3 are discussed. In advanced gastric cancer the incidence of microscopic metastases in the paraaortic lymph nodes is 6% to 33% (Takashima & Kosaka, 2005). Since 1980s superextended lymph node dissection is carried out in specialized centers in Japan. The Japanese Clinical Oncology Group conducted a randomized trial comparing D2 and D2 plus paraaortic lymphadenectomy among patients with curable gastic cancer (Sasako et a., 2008). The overall morbidity was 24% and even though the mobidity was higher in the D2 plus group it did not significantly differ. (28% vs 21%). There was no difference in hospital mortaliy between the two groups as well overall survival after 5 years. The blood loss and operation time are signifiantly increased in the D2 plus paraaortic lymph node dissection group (Sano et al., 2004).

The rationale behind D4 resecion is that to obtain a safe dissection margin for the lymph node involvement in the N2 and N3 stations. It is proposed that when the D-number is greater than the N-number, recurrence can be decreased. Accordingly, D2 gastrectomy is effective for N1 patients. In this sense, D4 dissection has been considered to improve the survival of patients with N2 or N3 involvement. D4 dissection had been practiced at many Asian institutions and Asian surgeons have proposed D4 dissection as a surgical technique to remove micrometastasis in the No. 16 lymph node. Micrometastasis in No. 16 lymph nodes was detected in 20% to 31% of patients with advanced gastric cancer, who underwent curative gastrectomy (Yonemura et al., 2008).

The major lymphatic channels from the upper half of the stomach run along the left gastric artery (No. 7), posterior gastric artery (No. 11), and splenic artery. In contrast, lymphatic channels from the lower half of the stomach run along not only the common hepatic artery (No. 8) but also along the root of the superior mesenteric artery (No. 14). Efferent lymphatic channels from these nodes drain into the No. 16 nodes, which are named No. 16 a2 and No.16 b1. Accordingly, No. 16 a2 and No. 16 b1 are considered as the terminal nodes of the stomach. Cancer cells released from the N2 or N3 lymph node stations are trapped in the lymph nodes located in the bilateral space around the aorta (No. 16 a2-lateral, -pre, and -inter), before the systemic spreading of cancer cells through the thoracic duct. According to the literature, the 5-year survival rates of N4 patients who underwent D4 resection ranged from 14% to 30% (Yonemura et al., 2008). Neither JCOG tiral and nother east asian trial did not reveal any significant difference in survival between two groups(Sano et al., 2004; Yonemura et al., 2008). There has been a recent study from Poland that compares the two methods revealing that there was no difference in morbidity and mortality but survival yet remains to be analysed (Kulig et al. 2007).

However, a study from Italy on superextended lymphadectomy with a pouplation of 286 patients, even though it is not a randomized study but a review of cases between 1993 and 2007, reveal some long term survival chance for both pN3 and M1a patients, 31% and 17% respectively. There is also remarkably high survival rate in pN2 and pN3 subsets when no serosal invasion was demonstrated, reaching upto 60%. The authors of this study, (Roviello et al.) has some points on the previous studies carried out in Japan. The overall survival rates (5-year survival: 70%) in east asian studies are at least better by one third than those reported by specialized Western centres in advanced forms. The adopted lymphadenectomy in D2 group included third level nodes (posterior hepatic artery nodes, posterior hepatoduodenal ligament nodes, etc.) in tumour with antral location that lead to a 'D3 lymphadenectomy minus paraaortic nodes (PAN) dissection'. The extent of lymphadenectomy is indeed demonstrated by the extremely high number of removed nodes (mean: 53 for D2 and 73 for D2 plus paraaortic). Cases in which macroscopic involvement of PANs was evident at surgery were excluded from the study. As stated by the authors themselves, the percentage of involvement was lower than expected (8%) and the potential survival benefit possibly weakened. Furthermore, the post hoc subgroup analysis based on pathologic N and T stages showed a better survival rate in the D2 plus para-aortic group for patients without nodal involvement and for patients with tumour invasion limited to the subserosal layer (less than pT3). An extremely high chance of cure was observed in patients with tumors not involving the serosa (pT2) or absence of nodal metastases (pN0), even if survival probability did not reach the results of the Japanese trial. Particularly, long-term results were remarkable in pT2 N2 and N3 patients. One could speculate that in these particular subsets of patients, where the local control of the disease is essential, D3 lymphadenectomy may be of value in improving long-term results. On the contrary, in serosally exposed neoplasms, which are particularly prone to peritoneal dissemination, the extent of lymphadenectomy might not provide a survival advantage with respect to more limited dissection (Roviello et al., 2010) .

As a consequence the NCNN guide does not recommend D2 plus paraaortic lymph node dissection for patients with curable gastric cancer (T2b, T3 or T4).

3.4 Conclusion

The NCCN 2010 guideline states that in west the D2 resection is a recommended but not a required operation. Modified lymphadectomy without pancreaticosplenectomy is associated with low mortality and morbidity as well as with reasonable survival times when performed in institutions with sufficient experience in operative and postoperative management. While in the east standard surgery is D2 lymphadenectomy and so far has proved longer 5 year survival and less locoregional recurrence rates. Finally, in our study although extensive dissection had an increased morbidity, there was no significant statistical difference between the D1 and D2 procedures (Yuksel et al., 2009). As a conclusion, we think that D2 dissection can be carried out with safety in centers with experience.

4. Sentinel lymph node dissection

Sentinel node is the first lymph node that receives the drainage from primary tumor. A sentinel biopsy for gastric cancer is an intra operative diagnostic tool to detect lymph node metastasis (Ishii et al., 2008). The sentinel node hypothesis states that the histopathologic status of the first node on the lymphatic drainage pathway from a primary tumor reflects the tumor status of the entire lymphatic drainage basin . Underlying this hypothesis is the assumption that the surgeon can correctly and consistently identify this node(Hsueh et al., 2001).

The history of sentinel lymph node mapping dates back to 1977. Cabanas described and used the technique of lymphangiograms in patients with penile carcinoma (Cabanas, 1977). Later it gained more common use in the treatment of malignant melanoma and breast cancer. For epithelial tumors lymphatic spread is a common route of metastasis and the nodal status is important for staging and therefore in planning the surgical and adjuant therapies. Nodal involvement in gastric cancer depends on the depth of invasion and it is between 2-18% for tumors limited with mucosa or submucosa, and around 50 % for tumors which has invaded muscularis propria or subserosa, T1 and T2 respectively. Therefore in some cases there is a chance of resecting more tissue than what may be required. Given the high morbidity rates associated with extended dissections in elderly population and in general, especially in western countries, when compared to more limited dissections, alternative treatments to avoid the risks associated with this procedure has been discussed among surgeons. D2 lymph node dissection may be unnecessary for patients without lymph node metastasis (Cozzaglio et al., 2011). To decrease the perioperative morbidity and

mortality and to improve the quality of life, less invasive surgery has been employed on patients with node-negative gastric cancer. However, it is difficult to precisely diagnose lymph node metastasis using preoperative examinations such as endoscopic ultrasonography and computed tomography (Li et al., 2008).
Miwa et al. (2001) demonstrated that extended lymphadenectomy in patients with early gastric cancer (EGC) resulted in a significantly lower 10-year recurrence rate than limited lymph node dissection (D1). Among node-positive patients, the recurrence rate following D2 was significantly lower than that after D1. Among node-negative patients, there was no difference in recurrence rate between two groups. Based on these observations he suggested that there are two optimal methods of node dissections in EGC surgery based on nodal status. He further stated that sentinel node concept is important to understand nodal status and introduced the sentinel node concept to gastric area. In 34 of 35 patients, metastatic nodes were located along the lymphatic basins. Among them, 15 patients had metastasis only in the sentinel lymph nodes. Of 5 gastric lymphatic basins, 42% of the patients had involvement of one, 47% 2, and 12% 3. These results show that each EGC has its own lymphatic basins in which metastasis can develop. The more numbers of the sections there are, the higher the likelihood of nodal metastasis. This means that each frozen section slice carries the risk of being false negative. Therefore we should always dissect the lymphatic basins even in cases with no sentinel node metastasis. In addition, patients with sentinel nodes containing metastasis should be treated with the D2 procedure (Miwa et al., 2001).
The current Japanese guideline recommendations for early cancers that are seemingly lymph node negative are as follows:
For Stage IA (T1N0) tumors Endoscopic Mucosal Resection EMR or modified gastrectomy (MG) is indicated according to the following instruction.

Depth of invasion	Histology	Size	Indication
Mucosa(M)	differentiated	2cm	EMR
Mucosa(M)	else		MG A
Submucosa(SM)	differentiated	1.5cm	MG A
Submucosa(SM)	else		MG B

Table 2. Treatment indication for Stage IA

EMR should be indicated to patients with small mucosal cancer with no lymph node metastasis. The JGSA database suggests that intestinal type mucosal cancer less than 2cm in diameter has no lymph node metastasis. En-bloc resection is preferable because of risk of residual cancer left behind EMR, and 2cm is the upper limit of en-bloc resection. Then, accurate assessment of the depth of wall invasion, histological type and size of tumor is mandatory before carrying out EMR. Mucosal cancer that does not meet this condition should be treated by MG A. MG A is also indicated to the differentiated submucosal cancer less than 1.5 cm in diameter. Submucosal cancer that does not meet this condition should be treated by MG B. Type of gastrectomy is shown in Table 3.
The lymphatic basins are defined as the area containing the stained or radiologically marked lymphatic vessels and are divided into five categories according to the directions of arteries that surrounds the stomach as follows: the left gastric area, the right gastric area, the right gastroepiploic area, the left gastropeiploic are and the posterior gastric artery area.

Gastrectomy	Range of Resection	Dissection	Option
Modified A	< 2/3	D1 + No.7*	Vagus preserving
Modified B	< 2/3	D1 + No.7,8a,9	Pylorus preserving Laparoscopic
Standard	2/3	D2	
Extended	2/3	D2	D3
Combined resection			

*In case of lower third cancer, No.8a nodes should be dissected.
Standard gastrectomy includes proximal, distal or total gastrectomy associated with D2 dissection according to the size and location of the tumor.
The differentiated type: papillary, well and moderately differentiated tubular adenocarcinomas.
The undifferentiated type: poorly differentiated adenocarcinoma, mucinous adenocarcinoma and signet-ring cell adeno-carcinoma.

Table 3. Type of gastrectomy

A preoperative endoscopic injection of dye or radioactive tracer followed by intraoperative mapping, intraoperative endoscopic injection, intraoperative subserosal injection of dye are the the usual ways of defining the lymphatic basin. The injections are carried out in four quadrants of the tumor either by endoscopy or by open surgery. The dye guided method is safe convenient and cost-effective. The radioguided method is more costly and may confront legal issues (Miyashiro et al., 2010).

The sentinel node (SN) concept has revolutionized the approach to the surgical staging of both melanoma and breast cancer, and these techniques can yield patient benefit by avoiding various complications due to unnecessary prophylactic regional lymph node dissection in cases with negative SN for cancer metastasis. Clinical application of SN mapping for early gastric cancer had been controversial for years. However, single institutional results of SN mapping for early gastric cancer are almost acceptable results in terms of detection rate and accuracy to determine lymph node status. Hypothesizing that SN mapping plays a key role to obtain individual information and allows modification of the surgical procedure for early gastric cancer, The Japan Society of Sentinel Node Navigation Surgery (JSNNS) has conducted a prospective multicenter trial of SN mapping by a dual tracer method with radioactive colloid and blue dye. Between September 2004 and March 2008, 433 patients with early gastric cancer were accrued at 12 comprehensive hospitals. Patients were enrolled under JSNNS and each institutional review board-approved protocols. Eligibility criteria were that patients had clinically T1N0M0 or T2N0M0 single tumor with diameter of primary lesion less than 4cm without any previous treatments. Technetium-99m tin colloid and isosulfan blue were utilized as dual tracers for SN mapping. SN mapping was performed for 397 patients with early gastric cancer. Detection rate of hot and/or blue node using their procedure was 97.5% (387/397). The mean number of sentinel nodes per case was 5.6. Fifty-three of 57 cases with lymph node metastasis showed positive sentinel nodes. The sensitivity to detect metastasis based on SN status was therefore 93% in their experience. Accuracy of metastatic status based on SN was 99% (383/387). In two of the four SN false-negative cases, the tumor involved to pT2, and only one case showed the metastatic lymph node beyond the SN basin (Kitagawa et al., 2009). Reviewing the relevant data, it becomes evident that the success rate of SLN mapping varies from as high as 99% in the Hiratsuka et al. series or 95% in the Aikou et al. series to as low as 74% in other series.

4.1 Pertinent issues

Skip metastasis is defined as the detection of metastatically infiltrated extragastric lymph nodes (level 2) in the absence of perigatric lymph node (level 1) involvement (Lee et al., 2009). However, the existence of skip metastases maybe as high as 17% and because of the complex and multi directional status of the gastric lymphatic drainage and the alteration of lymphatic pathways in advanced tumors because of the obstruction caused by tumor deposits (Griniatsos et al., 2009). There are also concerns about the negative predictivity of the technique. In patients with histologically classified as level one lymph node negative early gastric cancer, micrometastatically infiltrated level 2 lyph nodes are detected in 10 % (Morgagni et al., 2003). The lymphatic drainage route is patient-specific and lesion-specific in gastric cancer due to complicated lymphatic streams from the stomach. The most common channel for metastasis has been analyzed by subdividing the location of the tumor. For upper-thirds, the left gastric artery channel (Nos. 1, 3, 7) is the most common route. For the lower- and middle-third tumors, the left gastric artery channel and right gastroepiploic artery channel (No. 4and No. 6) are equally frequent routes. The following factors could play some role in the pathogenesis of skip metastasis: (1) Occult metastasis or micrometastasis to N1 nodes may have been missed during the dissection or routine histopathologic examination; (2) There may have been some aberrant lymphatic drainage patterns in patients with gastric cancer through which metastasis bypassed the lymphatic vessels; (3) Lymphatic flows to the N1 nodes may have been blocked by cancer tissue; (4) Free cancer cells may diffuse through regional nodes to distant nodes because the microenvironment in N1 nodes is unfit for the development of metastasis (Li et al., 2008)

In overweight patients when the cancer is located in the upper third of the stomach dense fat can conceal the visualization of SNL. When harvested lymph nodes are smaller than 3 false negativity increases. So maybe instead of lymph node biopsy, limited lymphadenectomy or lymphatic basin dissection may lead to better results. This is not actually a sentinel node biopsy because it is not a single pick biopsy but a limited resection. However if there are too many lymph nodes in the sentinel piece it will be hard to examine by frozen section.

When a lymph node micrometastasis is identified, routine extended resection is indicated but currently it is hard to detect micrometastasis in a short time during the operation.Another shortcoming is that in cases where SNs dont contain metastasis how to determine the extent of dissection.

The presence of micrometastasis in a lymph node is a critical issue for the clinical application of sentinel node biopsy for gastric cancer. There has been found micrometastases among patients who had been classified as tumor-free in routine histological examination.

Micrometastases may be found by using step sectioning, immunohistochemical (IHC) staining and reverse transcriptase-polimerase chain reaction. Matsumoto et al. (2002) demonstrated that the reverse transcriptase chain reaction is more sensitive than IHC for detection of micrometastases. However Yamamoto et al. (2001) suggested that positive results with a molecular array may not be indicative of the presence of viable tumor cells but rather the presence of tumor dna thus may be associated with an increase rate of false positivity. The serial sectioning with IHC is thought to be the most accurate method for detection of lymph node micrometastases. In a study by Ishii et al. (2008) they demonstrated that the the sentinel nodes were the first to receive micrometastases and they found no micrometastasis without the sentinel lymph node metastasis. They also suggested that it is sufficient to examine the sentinel lymph node for micrometastasis to determine whether or not there are lymph node micrometastases in patients with gastric cancer. Ajisaka et al. have proposed that dissection of the lymph nodes in the same lymphatic basin with the SN maybe mandatory even if the SN does not contain metastasis. Afer they found out that mestastatic nonsentinel nodes lie within th same basin with micrometastatic SNs, they proposed that the dissection of lymphatic basin containing SNs is minimal requirement for early stage gastric cancer even for patients without histologically detectable metastases in SNs (Ajisaka et al., 2003).

Another issue is that the reports from far Asia yields and accuracy rate of 98%, whereas in Europe the false negativity increases as well as accuracy to drops to 80%. In a study from Tel Aviv University they concluded that while in T1 And T2 tumors sentinel node mapping may be of assistance in decision making process regarding the extent of lymphadenectomy, SLN mapping in patients with T3 tumors maybe misleading in a third of the patients and therefore is not advised (Rabin et al., 2010).

5. Micrometastases and early gastric cancer

While the presence of lymph node metastases in early gastric cancer (EGC) is the most significant prognostic factor, the relevance of lymph node micrometastases (MM) remains uncertain. In 1996 Maehara noticed that even after curative resection of an early gastric cancer, some patients die of a recurrence. It is thought that patients with early gastric cancer who died of their disease had occult micrometastases in perigastric lymph nodes at the time of the original diagnosis.

Saito et al. (2007) studied seven hundred and sixty-five patients with early gastric cancer who underwent curative gastrectomy and analyzed them to identify the prognostic factor. The recurrence was observed in 17 patients. Hematogenous recurrence was observed most frequently (47.1%), followed by peritoneal recurrence (23.5%). Of 17 patients with recurrence, 6 (35.3%) patients died more than 5 years after operation. The prognosis was poorer when the patients were older, and the depth of invasion was greater, lymph node metastasis, lymphatic involvement, and vascular involvement were present, and lymph node dissection was limited. The independent prognostic factors were lymph node metastasis, lymph node dissection, and age by multivariate analysis using Cox proportional hazards. Micrometastases within lymph nodes were confirmed in 3 of 6 node-negative patients with recurrence (Saito et al., 2007). Several other studies have also supported the poorer prognosis of occult metastasis in early gastric cancer patients. In retrospective studies the frequency of micrometastasis in early gastric cancer can be as high as 20% and in most studies they are associated with poorer survival and more recurrence.

In a study by Liang Cao et al. MM was significantly associated with tumor size and lymphatic invasion . The statistically significant prognostic factors affecting 5-year survival rates were depth of tumor invasion, tumor size, lymphatic invasion, MM, and type of MM. The presence of MM, and particularly the cluster-type MM ($P<0.001$), were independent prognostic factors in pN0 early gastric cancer patients : The incidence of lymph node MM in patients with node negative early gastric cancer was 21.3%, and cancer cell cluster type of MM proved a primary independent prognostic factor for pN0 early gastric cancer patients (Cao et al.,2011)

Many studies have proved that there are two types micrometastases in lymph nodes: single-cell type and clustered-cell type. This can be explained by invoking the concept of tumor cell dormancy. Studies report that single cancer cells in lymph nodes may be associated with cells either under cell-cycle arrest or approaching apoptosis. According to cancer stem cell theory, an alternative explanation is that the disseminated cancer cells in some of the patients arose from the spread of nontumorigenic cells and only when cancer stems cells disseminate, and subsequently self-renew, will metastatic tumors form. Cancer stem cell can proliferate and form clusters of tumor cells, and nontumorigenic cells form single cells lymph node MM. Only when cancer stem cells disseminate and self-renew will the cluster type of MM form. Cancer stem cell theory predicts that the prognosis of clustered-cell MM should be worse compared to single-cell MM.. The 5-year survival rate for the group of patients with cluster-type MM (45.8%) was significantly lower than that for the group with negative (92.9%) or single-cell MM (80%). Cluster type of MM was proved a major independent prognostic factor for histologically node negative gastric cancer patients. This phenomenon can be explained by the association of clustering with the presence true cancer stem cells (Cao et al., 2011). Cai describes that a high incidence of nodal involvement is found in submucosal cancers of large size (>2 cm; 43%), a depressed type (48%) and lymphatic invasion. A higher incidence of microinvasion is found with the diffuse-type carcinoma (33%) (Cai et al., 2000).

Morgagni et al. studied 5400 lymph nodes dissected from 300 patients treated surgically for EGC between 1976 and 1999, all of whom were histologically pN0. Micrometastases were defined as single or small clusters of neoplastic cells identifiable only by immunohistochemical methods. Lymph node micrometastases were observed in 30 of the 300 patients (10%). No significant correlation was observed between micrometastases and other clinicopathological characteristics. Analysis of overall survival showed no significant difference between positive or negative micrometastasis groups. The results of their study show that the presence of lymph node micrometastases in EGC does not influence patient prognosis (Morgagni et al., 2003).

6. Micrometastasis in locally advanced and advanced tumors

Giuli reviewed micrometastasis in gastric cancer in 2003. Nakajo et al. (2001) reported that lymph node micrometastasis was correlated with a significantly worse survival rate in patients with T1 or T2 tumors . Cai et al. (1999) also found a significant relationship between lymph node micrometastasis and poor prognosis in patients with T3 gastric cancer. However, Fukagawa et al. found that the presence of lymph node micrometastasis did not affect the survival in large numbers of patiens with T2 cancer (Fukagawa et al., 2001). To clarify the prognostic importance of lymph node micrometastasis in patients with gastric cancer, histologically node-negative gastric cancers invading the muscularis propria or deeper (T2 and T3) were selected by Yasuda. The author's results indicate that lymph node micrometastasis is an independent prognostic indicator for patients with histologically node-negative gastric cancer invading the muscularis propria or deeper (T2 or T3). Micrometastasis of four or more lymph nodes or micrometastasis of level 2 nodes was significantly associated with a poor outcome. Lymph node metastasis is linked to tumor progression. Lymph node micrometastasis in gastric cancer is also associated with deep invasion through the gastric wall, large tumor size, and positive lymphatic or venous invasion. In this study, although no relationship was found between the presence of lymph node micrometastasis and clinico-pathologic characteristics, a weak association was found between lymph node micrometastasis and depth of wall invasion. In this series, the most common pattern of recurrence was peritoneal and lung metastasis. Similar to these results, previous studies reported that lymph node micrometastasis was strongly associated with subsequent development of hematogenous and peritoneal metastases, but not locoregional lymph node recurrence (Yasuda et al., 2002). Cai et al. studied cases of pT3 gastric cancer and found out even when standard histological staining reveals no evidence of metastases in the regional lymph nodes, patients still may die of postoperative recurrence of the tumor. Evidence of occult involvement was found in 299 of 2310 (13%) lymph nodes and in 54 of 83 (65%) patients with pT3 gastric cancer. An analysis of survival demonstrated the limited 5-year survival of patients with occult involvement in their resected lymph nodes, as compared with that of patients without involvement. Moreover, the patients in whom group 2 lymph nodes had occult cancer cells had a significantly poorer prognosis than those in whom occult involvement was limited to group 1 lymph nodes (Cai et al., 1999) .

Lee et al. studied the overall 5-year survival rate of patients in the MM negative group (76%) was higher compared with the rate of patients in the MM positive group (49%) for both patients with EGC and patients with AGC (Table 4). The effect of MM was most pronounced among patients in the Stage I and LNM negative group . There was a significant correlation between MM and depth of tumor invasion. Patients with MM had a decreased 5-year survival rate (49%) compared with patients without MM (76%) for both early and advanced gastric carcinoma. The effect of MM on survival was most pronounced for patients in the Stage I and LNM negative group (Lee et al., 2002).

7. Early gastric cancer and lymphadenectomy

Early gastric cancer is a more common entity in the east where screening programs are active, In the west most of the cancers are locally advanced or advanced at the time of diagnosis at present. The outcome of surgical treatment for early gastric cancer is satisfactory. Early gastric cancer is limited to mucosa or submucosa with or without lymph node metastasis. Even though the surgical treatment has excellent results in the management of early gastric cancer, the presence of lymph node metastasis is the most important prognostic factor.

For intramucosal cancer lesions with a differentiated histological type and without lymphatic-vascular involvement or ulcerative findings within the cancerous lesion there is a minimal risk for lymph node invasion. The surgical treatment is excellent even in lymph node positive diease. In a study by Sano et al. in which they summarized their findings in 1475 patients and reviewed 20 other articles in Japan about early gastric cancer, they pointed out that recurrence was higher in submucosal group (2,6%) than in mucosal grup (0,4%) and in lymph node positive group (7,3%) than the node free group (0,7%). In addition to this, histologically well differentiated tumors tended to recur more. The modes of recurrence were lymphatic, hematogenous, local peritoneal or a combination of these (Sano et al., 1993)

In their literature review they found out the overall recurrence rate was between 0,25% and 4,18% with a mean of 1,9%. The principal route of recurrence which led to death was hematogenous route in 59,3% of the patients and 68% of these recurrent tumors were well differentiated. Nevertheless, all the papillary carcinomas and five out of six poorly differentiated adenocarcionomas that recurred had positive lymph nodes at the time of diagnosis. The recurrence modes were almost similar for both nodal and node-free diseases, hematogenous recurrence being the most prominent one. As a conclusion, submucosal invasion, node positivity, histologically differentiated tumors and type 2a and 2c are high risk group. Traditional surgical resection is associated with 90% survival over 10 years (Sano et al., 1993).

Although there was a controversy on the extent of lymph node dissection in the past, today there is a concensus that limited D1 dissection is suitable for most of the cases. The reason for a minimally invasive treatment is the low incience of lymp node metastasis. Only 2% (range 0-4,8%) of patients with mucosal cancer will have positive lymph nodes. However when the tumor invades the submucosa this rate is about %20 (range15-25%) and this metastasis is not confined to the first lympatic echelon, especially when the submucosal lesion is bigger than 2 cms in diameter (Roukos et al., 2002).

For tumors which have exceeded the mucosa the risk factors for lymph node metastasis are tumor size larger than 30 mm, undifferentiated histologial type, lymphatic vascular involvement and submucosal invasion more than 0,5 mm. Additional surgery with lymph node dissection is of little benefit for tumors that satisfy the following conditions. No lymphovascular involvement, tumor size smaller than 2 cm, differentiated histological tpe and depth of submucosal penetrations smaller than 0,5mm.

According to the Japanese guideline 2004 for macroscopic mucosal cancer of differentiated type (papilary, tubuler carcinoma grade1, tubullary carcinoa gade 2) less than 2 cm in diameter with no ulceration or scar in cases of depressed type, irrespective of macroscopic type, no lymph node dissection is recommended. In such cases local excision of tumor with endoscopic procedures are considered sufficient if the procedure is carried out in a specialized center. For T1 cancers which are not indicated for EMR and which are with little possibility of lymph node metastasis, are expected to be cured with D1+α dissection. Such conditions are macroscopic mucosal cancer (more than 21 mms) without lymph node metastasis and macroscopic submucosal cancer of differentiated type less than 1.5 cm in diameter without lymph node metastasis . An α dissection refers to dissection of first echelon lymph nodes and the 7th lymp node station in the second tier with addition of the 8th nodal station in cancers of the lower third with standard gastrectomy that is removal of two thirds of stomach. If that the cancer is differentiated type, ≤ 2.0 cm in diameter, no ulceration in cases of depressed-type and there is involvement of the first tier of lymph nodes modified or if the submucosal cancer is differentiated type but more than 1,5 cms without lymph node involvement surgery-B (subtotal gastrectomy with the removal of first tier lymph nodes as well as lymph node stations 7, 8a, 9) is recommended. For other T1 tumors up to N2 nodal involvement standard surgery that is subtotal gastrectomy with the removal of second tiers of nodes is recommended. A very careful pre and intraoperative assesment of lymph nodes are mandatory and in case of any suspicion standard gastrectomy should be carried out.

8. References

Adachi, Y.; Oshiro, T. & Mori, M., et al. (1997). Tumor size as a simple prognostic indicator for *gastric* carcinoma. *Ann Surg Oncol*, Vol.4, No.2, (March 1997), pp: 137-40, ISSN 1068-9265

Aikou, T.; Kitagawa, Y. & Kitajima, M., et al. (2006). Sentinel lymph node mapping with GI cancer. *Cancer Metastasis Rev*. Vol.25, No.2, (June 2006), pp. 269-77, ISSN 0167-7659

Ajisaka, H. & Miwa, K. (2003) Micrometastases in sentinel nodes of gastric cancer. *Br J Cancer*, Vol.89, No.4, (August 2003), pp.18676-80, ISSN 0007-0920

Akajo, A.; Natsugoe, S. & Ishigami, S., et al. (2001). Detection and prediction of micrometastasis in the lymph nodes of patients with pN0 gastric cancer. *Ann Surg Oncol,* Vol.8, No.2, (March 2001), pp. 158-62, ISSN 1068-9265

Ajisaka H, Miwa K. Micrometastases in sentinel nodes of gastric cancer. Br J Cancer. 2003 Aug 18;89(4):676-80. PubMed PMID: 12915877; PubMed Central PMCID:PMC2376932.

Arigami, T.; Natsugoe, S.& Uenosono, Y., et al. (2006). Evaluation of sentinel node concept in gastric cancer based on lymph node micrometastasis determined by reverse transcription-polymerase chain reaction. *Ann Surg.* (March 2006) Vol.243, No.3. pp.341-47, ISSN 0003-4932

Bando, E.; Yonemura, Y; & Taniguchi, K., et al. (2002). Outcome of ratio of lymph node metastasis in gastric carcinoma. *Ann urg Oncol,* Vol.9, No.8, (October 2002), pp. 775–84 ISSN, 1068-9265

Biondi, A.; Persiani, R. & Cananzi, F., et al. (2010). R0 resection in the treatment of gastric cancer: Room for improvement. *World J Gastroenterol,* Vol.16, No. 27, (July 2010), pp. 3358–70, ISSN 1007-9327

Bonenkamp, JJ.; Songun I. & Hermans, J., et al. (1995). Randomised comparison of morbidity after D1 and D2 dissection for gastric cancer in 996 Dutch patients. *Lancet.* Vol.345, No.8952, (March 1995), pp. 745-48, ISSN 0140-6736

Bonenkamp JJ., Hermans, J. & Sasako, M., et al. (1998). Quality control of lymph node dissection in the Dutch randomized trial of D1 and D2 lymph node dissection for gastric cancer. *Gastric Cancer,* Vol.1, No.2, (March 1998), pp.152-59, ISSN 1436-3291

Bonenkamp, JJ.; Hermans, J. & Sasako, M., et al. (1999). Dutch Gastric Cancer Group. Extended lymph-node dissection for gastric cancer. *N Engl J Med,* Vol.340, No.12, (March 1999), pp. 908-14, ISSN 0028-4793

Cabanas RM. . (1977). An approach for the treatment of penile carcinoma. *Cancer,* Vol.39, No.2, (February 1977), pp. 456-66 , ISSN 0008-543X

Cai, J.; Ikeguchi, M. & Maeta, M., et al. (1999). Clinicopathological value of immunohistochemical detection of occult involvement in pT3N0 gastric cancer. *Gastric Cancer,* Vol.2, No.2, (August 1999), pp. 95-100, ISSN 1436-3291 (Electronic)

Cai, J.; Ikeguchi, M. & Maeta, M., et al. (2000). Micrometastasis in lymph nodes and microinvasion of the muscularis propria in primary lesions of submucosal gastric cancer. *Surgery.* Vol.127, No.1, pp.32-9, (January 2000), ISSN 0039-6060

Cao, L. Hu, X,. & Zhang, Y., et al. (2011). Adverse prognosis of clustered cell versus single-cell micrometastases in pN0 early gastric cancer. *J Surg Oncol,* Vol.103, No.1, (January 2011), pp. 53-6, ISSN 096-9098 (Electronic)/0022-4790 (Linking)

Cai, J.; Ikeguchi, M. & Maeta, M. (2000). Micrometastasis in lymph nodes and microinvasion of the muscularis propria n rimary lesions of submucosal gastric cancer. *Surgery,* Vol.127, No.1, (January 2000), pp. 32-9, ISSN 0039-6060

Coburn, NG. (2009). *Lymph nodes and gastric cancer. Journal of Surgical Oncology,* Vol. , No.4, (March 2009), pp: 199–206, ISSN 1096-9098 (Electronic)/ 0022-4790 (Linking)

Cozzaglio, L.; Bottura, R. & Di Rocco, M. (2011). Sentinel lymph node biopsy in gastric cancer: possible applications and limits. *Eur J Surg Oncol,* Vol.37, No.1, (January 2011), pp.55-9, ISSN 0748-7983

Csendes, A.; Burdiles, & Rojas. J., et al. (2002). A prospective randomized study comparing D2 total gastrectomy versus D2 total gastrectomy plus splenectomy in 187 patients with gastric carcinoma. *Surgery* , Vo.131, No.4, (April 2002), pp. 401- 7, ISSN 0039-6060

Cuschieri, A.; Weeden, S. & Fielding, J., et al. (1999). Patient survival after D1 and D2 resections for gastric cancer: long-t erm results of the MRC randomized surgical trial. Surgical Co-operative Group. *Br J Cancer,* Vol.79, No.9-10, (March 1999), pp.1522-30, ISSN 0007-0920

Díaz de LA.; Yarnoz, C. & Aguilar, R., et al. (2008). Rationale for gastrectomy with D2 lymphadenectomy in the treatment of gastric cancer. *Gastric Cancer,* Vol.11, No.2, (July 2008), pp.96-102, ISSN 1436-3291

de Gara, CJ.; Hanson, J. & Hamilton, S. (2003). A population-based study of tumor-node relationship, resection margins, and surgeon volume on gastric cancer survival. *Am J Surg* , Vol.186, No.1, (July 2003), pp. 23-27, ISSN 0002-9610

Degiuli, M.; Sasako, M. & Ponti, A., et al. Survival results of a multicentre phase II study to evaluate D2 gastrectomy for gastric cancer. *Br J Cancer,* Vol.90, No.9, (May 2004), pp.1727-32, ISSN 0007-0920

Dicken, BJ.; Bigam, DL. & Cass C. (2005). Gastric adenocarcinoma: review and considerations for future directions. *Ann Surg.* ; vol.241, No.1, (January 2005), pp. 27–39, ISSN: 0003-4932/05/24101-002

Dikken, JL.; Jansen, Epp. & Cats, A., et al. (2010). Impact of the extent of surgery and postoperative chemoradiotherapy on recurrence patterns in gastric cancer. *J Clin Oncol,* Vol.28. No.14, (May 2010), pp. 2430-6 ISSN 1527-7755 (Electronic)/0732-183X (Linking)

Siegwart, R. (2001). Indirect Manipulation of a Sphere on a Flat Disk Using Force Information. *International Journal of Advanced Robotic Systems,* Vol.6, No.4, (December 2009), pp. 12-16, ISSN 1729-8806

Fukagawa, T.; Sasako, M. & Mann, GB., et al. Immunohistochemically detected micrometastases of the lymph nodes in patients with gastric carcinoma. *Cancer,* Vol.92, No.4, (August 2001), p.753-60, ISSN 0008-543X

Ganpathi, IS.; So, JBY. & Ho, KY., et al. (2006). Endoscopic ultrasonograpy for gastric cancer. *Surg Endosc,* Vol.20, No.4, (April 2006), pp. 559–562 ISSN 1432-2218 (Electronic)/ 0930-2794 (Linking)

Giuli, R. http://www.Surgical Oncology.net ISSN 1591-1063

Griniatsos, J.; Gakiopoulou, H. & Yiannakopoulou E., et al. (2009).Routine modified D2 lymphadenectomy perfor- mance in pT1-T2N0 gastric cancer.*World J Gastroenterol,* Vol.15, No.44, (November 2009), pp. 5568-5572 ISSN 1007-9327

Gunderson, LL. & Sosin, H. (1982). Adenocarcinoma of the stomach: Area of failure in a re-operation series (second or symptomatic look) clinicopahtologic correlation and implications for adjuvant therapy. *Int J Radiat Oncol Biol Phys* Vol.8, No.1, (January 1982), ppp. 1-11, ISSN 0360-3016

Gunderson LL. (2002).Gastric cancer--patterns of relapse after surgical resection. *Semin Radiat Oncol,* Vol.12, No.2, (April 2002), pp.150-61, ISSN 1053-4296

Hartgrink, HH.; van de Velde, CJ. & Putter. H., et al. (2004). Extended lymph node dissection for gastric cancer: who may benefit? Final results of the randomized Dutch gastric cancer group trial. *J Clin Oncol* (2004); Vol.22, No.11, (June 2004), pp: 2069-77, ISSN 0732-183X

Herrera, L. & Villareal, JR. (1992). Incidence of metastases from rectal adenocarcinoma in small lymph nodes detected by a clearing technique. *Dis Colon Rectum,* Vol.35, No.8, (August 1992), pp. 783-788 ISSN 0012-3706

Hiratsuka, M.; Miyashiro, I. & Ishikawa, O., et al. (2001). Application of sentinel node biopsy to gastric cancer surgery. *Surgery,* Vol.129, No.3, (March 2001), pp. 335-40 ISSN 0039-6060

Hsueh, EC.; Roderick, RT. & Giuliano, AE., et al. (2001). *Lymphoscintgraph and lymphatic mapping for identification of sentinel lymph nodes. World J Surg, (June 2001). Vol.25, No.6,pp. 794-797 ISSN 0364-2313*

Hundahl, SA; Phillips, JL & Menck, HR. (2000) The National Cancer Data Base Report on poor survival of US gastric carcinoma patients treated with gastrectomy: fifth edition American Joint Committee on Cancer staging, proximal disease, and the 'different disease' hypothesis. *Cancer* , vol.88, No.4, (February 2000), pp. 921–932. ISSN 0008-543X

Huhndahl, SA. (2002). Staging, migration, and patterns of spread in gastric cancer. *Seminars in Radiation oncology.* Vol. 12, No.2, (April 2002), pp. 141-149 ISSN 1053-4296

Hundahl SA. (2006), Low maruyama index surgery for gastric cancer. *Scand J Surg.,* Vol.95, No.4, (2006), pp. 243-8. ISSN 1457-4969

Hundahl, SA.; Peeters, KC. & Kranenbarg, EK., et al. (2007). Improved regional control and survival with "low Maruyama Index" surgery in gastric cancer: autopsy findings from the Dutch D1-D2 Trial. *Gastric Cancer.* June 2007, Vol.10, No.2 pp. 84-6 ISSN 1436-3291

Ishii, K.; Kinami, S. & Funaki, K., et al. (2008). Detection of sentinel and non-sentinel lymph node micrometastases by complete serial sectioning and immunohistochemical analysis for gastric cancer. J *Exp Clin Cancer Res,* 2008 May Vol.30 No.27, (May 2008), pp. 7. ISSN 1756-9966 (Electronic)/ 0392-9078 (Linking)

Ishikawa, S.; Shimada, S, & Miyanari, N., et al.(2009).Pattern of lymph node involvement in proximal gastric cancer. *World J Surg,* Vol.33, No.8, (August 2009), pp. 1687-92, ISSN 1432-2323(Electronic)/0364-2313 (Linking)

Japanese Gastric Cancer Society. Guidelines for Diagnosis and Treatment of Carcinoma of the Stomach. April 2004.

Kitagawa, Y.; Kubota, T & Kumai, K, et al. (2005) [Recent studies of sentinel lymph node. Multicenterprospective clinical trials of SN biopsy for gastric cancer]. *Gan To Kagaku Ryoho,* Vol.32, No.5, (May 2005) pp. 695-8 ISSN 0385-0684.

Kitagawa, Y.; Takeuchi, H. & Takagi, Y., et al. (2009). Prospective multicenter trial of sentinel node mapping for gastric cancer. *Journal of Clinical Oncology,* 2009 ASCO Annual Meeting Proceedings (Post-Meeting Editition), Vol.27, No.15S (May 20 Supplement 2009), pp.4518

Kim, HJ; Karpeh, MS. & Brennan MF. (2001). Standardization of the extent of lymphadenectomy for gastric cancer: impact on survival. *Advances in Surgery,* volume 35 (2001), pp. 203-223, ISSN 0065-3411

Kitamura, K.; Nishida, S. & Ichikawa, D., et al. (1999). No survival benefit from combined pancreaticosplenectomy and total gastrectomy for gastric cancer. *Br J Surg* , Vol.86, No.1, (January 1999), pp. 119 –122 ISSN 0007-1323

Kodera, Y.; Yamamura, Y. & Shimizu, Y., et al. (1997). Lack of benefit of combined pancreaticosplenectomy in D2 resection for proximal-third gastric carcinoma. *World J Surg* , Vol.21, No.6, (July-August 1997), ppp. 222– 627 ISSN 0364-2313

Kodera, Y.; Yamamura, Y. & Shimizu, Y., et al. (1998). *Lymph node status*assessment for gastric carcinoma: is the number of metastatic lymph nodes really practical as a parameter for N categories in the TNM classification? *J Surg Oncol,* Vol.69 No.1,(September 1998), . 15–20 ISSN 0022-4790

Krijnen, pp.; den Dulk, M. & Meershoek-Klein Kranenbarg E., et al. Improved survival after resectable non-cardia gastric cancer in The Netherlands: the importance of surgical training and quality control. *Eur J Surg Oncol*Vol.35, No.7, (Jul 2009), pp. 715-20 ISSN 1532-2157 (Electronic)/0748-7983 (Linking)

Kulig, J.,; Popiela,T. & Kolodziejczyk, P., et al. (2007). Polish Gastric Cancer Study Group. Standard D2 versus extended D2 (D2+) lymphadenectomy for gastric cancer: an interim safety analysis of a multicenter, randomized, clinical trial. *Am J Surg,* Vol.193, No.1, (January 2007), pp.10-5, ISSN 1879-1883 (Electronic)/ ISSN 0002-9610 (Linking)

Lee, E.; Chae, Y. & Kim, I., et al. (2002). Prognostic relevance of immunohistochemically detected lymph node micrometastasis in patients with gastric carcinoma. *Cancer,* Vol.94, No.11, (June 2002), pp.2867-73, ISSN 0008- 543X

Lee, SE.; Lee, JH. & Ryu, KW., et al. (2009). Sentinel node mapping and skip metastases in patients with early gastric cancer. *Ann Surg Oncol*. Vol.16, No.3, pp. 603-8 ISSN 1534-4681 (Electronic)/1068-9265 (Linking)

Li, C.; Kim, S. & Lai, JF., et al. (2008). Solitary lymph node metastasis in gastric cancer. *J Gastrointest Surg.* Vol.12, No.3 (March 2008), pp. 550-4 ISSN 1091-255X

MacDonald, J; Smalley, S & Benedetti, J., et al. Chemoradiotherapy after surgery compared with surgery alone for adenocarcinoma of the stomach or gastroesophageal junction. *N Engl J Med.* 2001; vol.345, No.10, (September 2001), pp. 725–729, ISSN 0028-4793

McCulloch, pp.; Nita, ME. & Kazi, H.(2004). *Extended versus limited lymph* nodes dissection technique for adenocarcinoma of the stomach. *Cochrane Database Syst Rev,* (October 2004) Vol.18, No.4, CD001964 ISSN 1469- 493X (Electronic)/1361-6137 (Linking)

Maehara, Y.; Orita, H. & Okuyama, T. (1992). Predictors of lymph node metastasis in early gastric cancer. *Br J Surg.* Vol.79, No.3, (March 1992), pp. :245-7 ISSN 0007-1323

Maehara, Y.; Oshiro, T, & Endo. K., et al. (1996). Clinical significance of occult micrometastasis lymph nodes from patients with early gastric cancer who died of recurrence. *Surgery*, Vol.119, No.4, (April 1996), pp.397-402, I SSN 0039-6060

Marchet, A.; Mocellin, S. & Ambrosi, A., et al. (2007). Italian Research Group for Gastric Cancer (IRGGC). The ratio between metastatic and examined lymph nodes (N ratio) is an independent prognostic factor in gastric cancer regardless of the type of lymphadenectomy: results from an Italian multicentric study in 1853 patients. *Ann Surg*. Vol.245, No.4, (April 2007), pp.543-52, ISSN 0003-4932

Marelli, D.; Roviello, F. & de Manzoni, G. (2002). Diffrent Patterns of Recurrence in Gastric Cancer Depending on Lauren's Histological Type: Longitudinal Study. *World Journal of Surgery,* Vol.26, No.9, (September 2002), pp. 1160-1165 ISSN 0364-2313

Maruyama, K.; Okabayashi, K. & Kinoshita, T. (1987). Progress in gastric cancer surgery in Japan and its limits of radicality. *World J Surg*. Vol.11, No.4, (August 1987), pp. 418-25 ISSN 0364-2313

Maruyama, K.; Gunven, pp. & Okabayashi, K., et al. (1989). Lymph node metastases of gastric cancer: general pattern in 1931 patients, *Ann Surg,* Vol.210, No.5, (November1989), pp: 596–602 ISSN 0003-4932

Maruyama, K.; Sasako, M. & Ki noshita T et al. (1995). Pancreas-preserving total gastrectomy for proximal gastric cancer. World J Surg, Vol.19 , No.4, (July-August 1995), pp 532–536 ISSN 0364-2313

Maruyama, K.; Sasako, M. & Kinoshita, T., et al. (1998) . Should systematic lymph node dissection be recommended for gastric cancer? *Eur J Cancer,* Vol.34, No.10, (September 1998), pp.1480-9, ISSN 0959-8049

Matsumoto, M.; Natsugoe, S. & Ishigami, S., et al. (2002). Lymph node micrometastasis and lymphatic mapping determined by reverse transcriptase-polymerase chain reaction in pN0 gastric carcinoma. *Surgery*. Vol. 131 N. 6, (June 2002), pp. 630-5 ISSN 0039-6060

Miwa K. (2001) [Optimal nodal dissection for early gastric cancer]. *Nippon Geka Gakkai Zasshi,* Vol.102, No.6, (June 2001), pp.484-9 ISSN 0301-4894

Miwa, K.; Kinami, S. & Taniguchi, K., et al. (2003). Mapping sentinel nodes in patients with early-stage gastric carcinoma. *Br J Surg,* Vol.90, No.2, (Feruary 2003), pp. 178-82 ISSN 0007-1323

Moriguchi, S.; Maehara. Y & Koenaga, D., et al. (1992). Risk factors which predict pattern of recurrence after curative surgery for patients with advanced gastric cancer. *Surgical Oncolgy* ,Vol.1, No.5, (October 1995), pp.341-346 ISSN 0960-7404

Morgagni, P.; Saragoni, L.& Scarpi, E., et al. (2003). Lymph node micrometastases in early gastric cancer and their impact on prognosis. *World J Surg,* Vol.27, No.5, (May 2003), pp. 558-61. ISSN 0364-2313

Morton, DL. & Bostick, PJ. (1999). Will the true sentinel node please stand? *Ann Surg Oncol* , (January-February 1999) vol.6, No.1 pp. 12- 4 ISSN 1068-9265

Nakajo, A.; Natsugoe, S. & Ishigami, S., et al. (2001. Detection and prediction of micrometastasis in the lymph nodes of patients with pN0 gastric cancer. *Ann Surg Oncol*. Vol.8, No.2, (March 2001), pp.158-62. ISSN 1068-9265

Nakamura, K.; Ueyama, T. & Yao, T,. et al. (1992). Pathology and prognosis of gastric carcinoma. Findings in 10,000 patients who underwent primary gastrectomy. *Cancer* , vol.70, No.5, (September 1992), pp. 1030-1037 ISSN 0008-543X

Peeters, KC., Hundahl, SA. & Kranenbarg, EK., et al. (2005). Low Maruyama index surgery for gastric cancer: blinded reanalysis of the Dutch D1-D2 trial. *World J Surg,* Vol.29, No.12, (December 2003), pp.1576-84 ISSN 0364-2313

Peeters, KC.; Kattan, MW. & Hartgrink, HH., et al. (2005). Validation of a nomogram for predicting disease-specific survivalafter an R0 resection for gastr ic carcinoma. *Cancer,* 1 Vol.103, No.4, (Feb 2005) pp. 702-7 ISSN 0008- 543X

Putter, H.; Sasako, M. & Hartgrink, HH., et al. Long-term survival with non-proportional hazards: results from the Dutch Gastric Cancer Trial. *Stat Med,* Vol. 24, No.18, (Sep 2005), pp. 2807-21 ISSN 0277-6715

Rabin, I.; Chikman, B. & Lavy, R., et al. (2010). The accuracy of sentinel node mapping according to T stage in patients with gastric cancer. *Gastric Cancer,* Vol.13, No.1, (March 2010), pp. :30-5 ISSN 0364-2313

Roviello, F.; Pedrazzani, C. & Marrelli, D., et al. (2010). Super-extended (D3) lymphadenectomy in advanced gastric cancer. *Eur J Surg Oncol,* Vol.36,No.5, (May 2010), pp.439-46, ISSN 1532-2157 (Electronic)/ 0748-7983 (Linking)

Roth, AD. (2003) Curative treatment of gastric cancer: towards a multidisciplinary approach? *Crit Rev Oncol Hematol,* Volume 46, Number 1, (April 2003), pp. 59-100, ISSN 1040-8428

Roukos, DH.; Fatouros, M. & Xeropotamos N., et al. (2002). Treatment of Gastric Cancer: Early-Stage, Advanced-Stage Cancer, Adjuvant Treatment .*Gastric Breast Cancer,* Vol.1, No.1, .(January –March 2002), pp.11-20, ISSN : 1109 - 7655

Saito H, Fukumoto Y & Osaki T et al. (2006) Distinct recurrence pattern and outcome of adenocarcinoma of the gastric cardia in comparison with carcinoma of other regions of the stomach.*World j surg* , Vol. 30, No.10, (October 2006), pp .1864-9 ISSN 0364-2313

Saito, H.; Osaki, T. & Murakami, D., et al. (2007). Recurrence in early gastric cancer--presence of micrometastasis in lymph node of node negative early gastric cancer patient with recurrence. *Hepatogastroenterology.* Vol.54, No.74, (March 2007), pp.620-4, ISSN 0172-6390

Sano, T.; Sasako, M. & Kinoshita, T., et al. (1993). Recurrence of early gastric cancer. *Cancer* Vol.72, No.11, (December 1993), pp. 3174-3178 ISSN 0008-543X

Sano, T.; Sasako, M. & Yamamoto, S.., et al. (2004). Gastric cancer surgery: morbidity and mortality results from a prospective randomized controlled trial comparing D2 and extended para-aortic lymphadenectomy--Japan Clinical Oncology Group study 9501. *J Clin Oncol.* 15 Vol.22, Vol.14, (July 2004), pp.2767-73 ISSN 0732-183X

Sasako, M.; McCulloch, P & Kinoshita, T., et al. (1995) New method to evaluate the therapeutic value of lymph node dissection for gastric cancer. *Br J Surg* , Vol.82, No.3, (March 1995), pp. 346 –351 ISSN 0007-1323

Sasako, M.; Saka, M. & Fukagawa, T., et al. Surgical treatment of advanced gastric cancer: Japanese perspective. *Dig Surg,,* Vol.24, No.2, (2007), pp.101-7 ISSN 0253-4886 (Print)/ 0253-4886 (Linking)

Sasako, M.; Sano, T. & Yamamoto, S., et al. (2008). Japan Clinical Oncology Group. D2 lymphadenectomy alone or with para-aortic nodal dissection for gastric cancer. *N Engl J Med,* Vol.359, No.5, (July 2008), pp.453-62, ISSN 1533-4406 (Electronic)/ 0028-4793 (Linking)

Schwarz, RE. & Smith, D. (2007). Clinical impact of lymphadenectomy extent in resectable gastric cancer of advanced stage. *Ann Surg Oncol,* (February 2007), Vol.14, No.2, pp. 317-28 ISSN 1068-9265

Shi, Y. & Zhou, Y. (2010). The role of surgery in the treatment of gastric cancer. *J Surg Oncol,* Vol.101, No.8, (June 2010), pp.687-92

Shin, SH.; Jung, H. & Choi SH., et al. (2009). The clinical significance of splenic hilar lymph node metastasis in proximal gastric cancer. *Ann Surg Oncol* , (May 2009), Vol. 16, No.5, ppp. 305-1309 ISSN 1534-4681 (Electronic)/1068-9 265 (Linking)

Shinohara, T.; Ohyama, S. & Yamaguchi, T., et al. Clinical value of multidetector row computed tomography in detecting lymph node metastasis of early gastric cancer. *Eur J Surg Oncol,* Vol.31, No.7, (September 2005) pp. 743–748 ISSN 0748-7983

Sierra, A.; Regueira, FM. & Hernández-Lizoáin, JL., et al. (2003). Role of the extended lymphadenectomy in gastric

cancer surgery: experience in a single institution. *Ann Surg Oncol.* 2003 Apr; Vol.10, No.3, (April 2003), pp.219-26, ISSN 1068-9265

Sivins,A .; Pedrazzani, C. & Roviello, F. (2009). Surgical treatment of gastric cancer in Latvia: results of centralized experience. *Eur J Surg Oncol,* Vol.35, No.5, (May 2009), pp. 481-5 ISSN 1532-2157 (Electronic)/0748-7983 (Linking)

Songun I I. & van de Velde CJ. (1996). Can Surgical Treatment Results in Gastric Cancer Be Improved? *Oncologist.* 1996 Vol.1, No.1&2, (1996) pp.36-40. ISSN 1549-490X (Electronic)/1083-7159 (Linking)

Songun, I.; Putter, H. & Kranenbarg, EM., et al. Surgical treatment of gastric cancer: 15-year follow-up results of the randomised nationwide Dutch D1D2 trial. *Lancet Oncol,* Vol.11, No.5, (2010 May), pp. 439-49 ISSN 1474-5488 (Electronic)/1470-2045 (Linking)

Smalley, SR.; Gunderson, L. & Teper, J., et al. (2002). Gastric surgical adjuvant radiotherapy consensus report: rationale and treatment implementation. *Int J Radiat Oncol Biol Phys.*,Vol.52, No.2), (February 2002), pp.283-93. ISSN 0360-3016

Takashima, S. & Kosaka, T. (2005). Results and controversial issues regarding a para-aortic lymph node dissection for advanced gastric cancer. Surg Today. Vol.35, No.4, 2005, pp.425-31, ISSN 0941-1291

Tanizawa, Y, & Terashima, M. (2010). Lymph node dissection in the resection of gastric cancer: Review of existing evidence. *Gastric Cancer* Vol.13, No.3, (August 2010), pp. 137-148, ISSN 1436-3291

Wagner, PK.; Ramaswamy, A. & Ruschoff, J., et al. (1991). Lymph node counts in the upper abdomen: Anatomic basis for lymphadenectomy in gastric cancer. *Br J Surg,* Vol. 78 No.7, (July 1991), ppp. 825-827 ISSN 0007-1323

Wu, CW.; Lo, SS. & Shen, KH. (2003) Incidence and factors associated with recurrence patterns after intended curative surgery for gastric cancer. *World J Surg.*, Vol.27, No.2, (February 2003), pp. 153-8 ISSN 0364-2313

Xu, DZ.; Geng, QR. & Long, Z.J, et al. (2009). Positive lymph node ratio is an independent prognostic factor in gastric cancer after d2 resection regardless of the examined number of lymph nodes. *Ann Surg Oncol ,* Vol.16, No.2, (February 2009), pp. 319–326 ISSN 1534-4681 (Electronic)/1068-9265 (Linking)

Yamamoto, H.; Miyake, Y. & Noura, S., et al.(2001) [Clinical significance of micrometastasis to lymph nodes in gastrointestinal tract cancers]. *Gan To Kagaku Ryoho,* Vol.28, No.6, (June 2001) , pp.776-83 ISSN 0385-0684

Yasuda, K.; Adachi, Y. & Shiraishi, N. (2002). Prognostic Effect of Lymph Node Micrometastasis in Patients With

Histologically Node-Negative Gastric Cancer. *Annals of Surgical Oncology,* Vol.9, No.8, (October 2002), pp. 771-4, ISSN 1068-9265

Yonemura, Y.; Wu ,CC. & Fukushima, N., et al. (2008). East Asia Surgical Oncology Group. Randomized clinical trial of D2 and extended paraaortic lymphadenectomy in patients with gastric cancer. *Int J Clin Oncol,* Vol.13, No.2, (April 2008), pp.132-7, ISSN 1341-9625

Yoon, SS. & Yang, HK. (2009) . Lymphadenectomy for Gastric Adenocarcinoma: Should West Meet East? The *Oncologist,* Vol. 14, No. 9, (September 2009), pp. 871-882, ISSN 1549-490X (Electronic)/1083-7159 (Linking)

Yoshida, M.; Ohtsu, A. & Boku, N., et al. (2004). Long-term survival and prognostic factors in patients with metastatic gastric cancers treated with chemotherapy in the Japan Clinical Oncology Group (JCOG) study. *Jpn J Clin Oncol,* Vol.34, no.11, (November 2004) pp.654-9, ISSN 0368-2811

Yu, W.; Choi, GS. & Chung, HY. (2006) Randomized clinical trial of splenectomy versus splenic preservation in patients with proximal gastric cancer. *Br J Surg* , Vol.93, No.5, (May 2006), pp. 559–563 ISSN 0007-1323

Yuksel, BC.; Ucar, NS. & Yildiz, Y., et al. (2009). Mide kanserinde standart D2 diseksiyona karşı D1 diseksiyonun mortalite ve morbidite çalışması. *Turkish Journal of Surgery ,* Vol.25, No.3, pp. 87-91 ISSN 1300-0705

Part 3

Chemotherapy

7

Prospective Study of Triple Combination Chemotherapy Consisting of Paclitaxel, S-1, and 24-Hour Infusion of Cisplatin (PSC) for Inoperable Highly Advanced Gastric Cancer

Kenji Ina[1], Ryuichi Furuta[1], Takae Kataoka[2], Satoshi Kayukawa[2] and Hiroaki Iwase[3]
[1]Department of Medical Oncology
[2]Department of Clinical Oncology
[3]Nagoya Memorial Hospital and Department of Gastroenterology
Nagoya Medical Center[5]
Nagoya,
Japan

1. Introduction

Although the prognosis of unresectable gastric cancer remains poor (Hohenberger & Gretshel, 2003), recent advances in chemotherapy for this cancer have considerably improved the therapeutic effects. An oral fluoropyrimidine anticancer agent, S-1, developed in Japan, was designed to enhance the anticancer activity of 5-FU via combination with two modulating substances: gimeracil to inhibit dihydropyrimidine dehydrogenase and potassium oxonate to reduce gastrointestinal toxicities (Shirasaka, et al, 1996). The antitumor effects of fluoropyrimidine are known to be enhanced through biochemical modulation of folate metabolism modified by cisplatin (Scanlon, et al, 1986), and combination therapy using S-1 and cisplatin reportedly achieves high response rates (Koizumi, et al, 2008 ; Lenz, et al, 2007). Therefore, in Japan, S-1 with cisplatin is the standard therapy for advanced gastric cancer. However, disease progression is still observed in up to 40% of cases (Iwase, et al, 2005; Koizumi, et al, 2008) and further improvement of treatment is thus necessary.

Taxanes have shown encouraging anti-tumor activities against various malignancies, including gastric cancer (Ohtsu, et al, 1998; Sulkes, et al, 1994). Taxane derivatives, docetaxel and paclitaxel, have a unique mechanism of action that differs from those of fluoropyrimidines and platinum compounds. The docetaxel containing combination regimens are associated with severe neutropenia (Yamaguchi, et al, 2006). Just recently, a phase I/ II study of docetaxel combined with S-1 plus cisplatin (DSC triple therapy) was conducted for advanced gastric cancer, and a very high tumor response rate was achieved with febrile neutropenia developing in approximately 20 % of patients (Nakayama, et al, 2008; Sato, et al, 2010). Paclitaxel combined with other drugs reportedly has tolerable toxicity (Kang, et al, 2008). In addition, continuous infusion of cisplatin for 24 hours has been used to minimize side effects including renal and hematological toxicity (Ina, et al, 2008; Iwase, et al, 2005) with anti-tumor effects the same as in previous reports (Koizumi, et al, 2008 ; Lenz, et al, 2007). Therefore, with the aim of improving the tumor response to S-1 plus cisplatin therapy, we combined paclitaxel with S-1 plus cisplatin (PSC triple therapy) for the treatment of advanced gastric cancer.

2. Patients and methods

Patients were eligible if they signed an informed consent document and met all of the following criteria; (1) pathologically proven inoperable gastric cancer and at least one measurable lesion; (2) age 20 to 75 years; (3) Eastern Cooperative Oncology Group performance status of 0 to 2; (4) white blood cell count between 4000 and 12,000 /mm^3, platelet count > 100,000/mm^3, haemoglobin > 8 g/ dl; serum bilirubin < 1.5 mg/ dl, aspartate aminotransferase and alanine aminotransferase < 3 times the upper limit of normal (ULN); and serum creatinin less than or equal to ULN; (5) no prior chemotherapy or one regimen that was completed > 4 weeks before entry. S-1 at a dose of 70 mg/m^2 was given orally twice daily for 2 weeks followed by 2 weeks rest. Paclitaxel at a dose of 120 mg/m^2 was administered by 2-hour infusion on day 1, cisplatin at a dose of 60 mg/m^2 by continuous infusion for 24 hours on day 14 (Figure 1). Patients received a maximum of 6 cycles. The objective response to chemotherapy was evaluated employing the criteria proposed by the Japanese Research Society for Gastric Cancer (Japanese Research Society for Gastric Cancer, 1995) for the primary lesion and according to RECIST (Response Evaluation Criteria in Solid Tumors) for metastatic lesions. A complete response (CR) was defined as the disappearance of all evidence of cancer for at least 4 weeks. According to RECIST, a partial response (PR) was defined as a greater than 50% tumor volume reduction. A new lesion or enlargement exceeding the original tumor size by 25% was defined as progressive disease (PD). All patients not in these categories were considered to have stable disease (SD). Progression-free survival (PFS) and overall survival (OS) were calculated from the start of PSC triple therapy until death or the most recent follow-up day. The Kaplan-Meier method was used to plot PFS and OS curves. The National Cancer Institute common toxicity criteria version 4.0 was applied to evaluate adverse effects Doses were adjusted at the initiation of subsequent cycles, if severe toxicity (grade 3 - 4) was present; S-1 was discontinued and then resumed at a reduced dose (10 mg/m^2/ day) and paclitaxel was reduced by 25% in the next cycle when toxicity resolved. Cisplatin was postponed until toxicity resolved; the maximum duration of postponement was no more than 2 weeks.

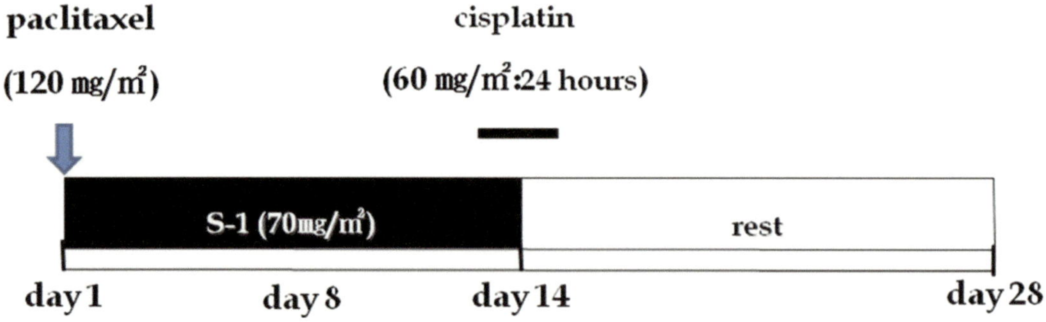

Fig. 1. PSC triple combination therapy

S-1 at a dose of 70 mg/m^2 was given orally twice daily for two weeks followed by two weeks rest. Paclitaxel at a dose of 120 mg/m^2 was administered by 2-hour infusion on day 1, cisplatin at a dose of 60 mg/m^2 by continuous infusion for 24 hours on day 15. Patients received a maximum of 6 cycles. Doses were adjusted at the initiation of subsequent cycles, if severe toxicity (grade 3–4) was present; S-1 was discontinued and then resumed at a reduced dose (10 mg/m^2/day) and paclitaxel was reduced by 25% in the next cycle when toxicity resolved. Cisplatin was postponed until toxicity resolved; the maximum duration of postponement was no more than 2 weeks.

3. Results

3.1 Study population

Ten patients with metastatic or recurrent gastric cancer were enrolled from November, 2005 to October, 2010 in our hospital. Patient characteristics are summarized in Table 1. There were 8 men and 2 women, with a median age of 65 (range, 57–73) years. Performance status was 0 in 4 patients, 1 in 2, and 2 in 4. Metastases were identified in the liver in 3 patients, the lung in 2, lymph nodes in 6, and the peritoneum in 7. Prior chemotherapy was conducted in 4 patients (S-1/ paclitaxel in 3; S-1 alone in 1), while the other 6 were chemo-naïve. These patients were administered a total of 40 cycles, with the median being 5 cycles (range, 3–6).

Characteristics		No. of patients
Gender		
	Male	8
	Female	2
Age		57 - 73
	Median	65
Performance Status		
	0	4
	1	2
	2	4
Pathology		
	Intestinal	4
	Diffuse	6
Target Lesions		
	Primary tumor	6
	Liver	3
	Lung	2
	Lymph nodes	6
	Peritoneum	7
	(Ascites)	(3)
Total cycles		3 - 6
	Median	5

Table 1. Patient backgrounds

3.2 Efficacy

The response rates according to site are shown in Table 2: primary lesion, 67% (4 of 6); lymph node metastases, 83% (5 of 6); liver metastases, 67% (2 of 3); and lung metastases, 100% (2 of 2). The overall response rate was 70% (7/10; CR 1, PR 6) and the disease control rate was 100%. Seven patients received subsequent chemotherapy: 3 S-1 alone, 3 S-1/irinotecan and, 1 paclitaxel alone. The median PFS was 373 days (95% CI: 160–573 days) (Figure 2). In this series, no patients underwent surgery after PSC, but the median OS was 747 days (95% CI: 488–1714 days) as shown in Figure 3.

	CR	PR	SD	PD	Response rate	CR rate
Overall	1	6	3	0	70 %	10 %
Primary lesion	1	3	2	0	67 %	10 %
Lymph node	1	4	1	0	83 %	10 %
Liver	0	2	1	0	67 %	0 %
Lung	1	1	0	0	100 %	50 %
Ascites	0	3	0	0	100 %	0 %

Table 2. Objective response rates

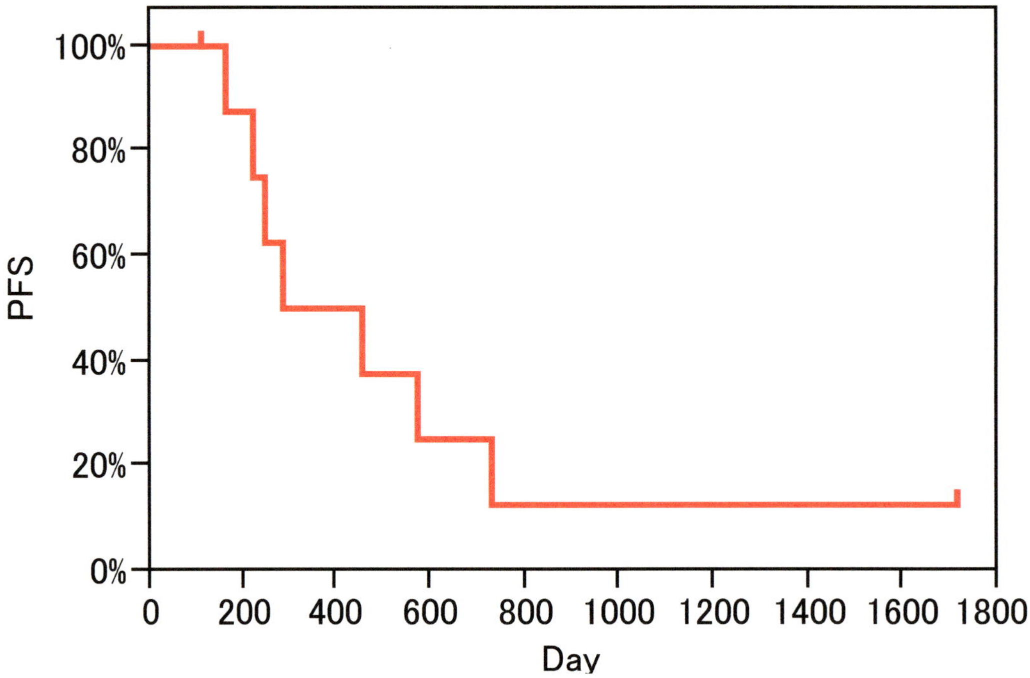

Fig. 2. Progression-free survival (PFS) in patients receiving PSC therapy
Kaplan-Meier analysis of PFS in 10 patients showed PFS to be 373 days (95% CI: 160–573 days).

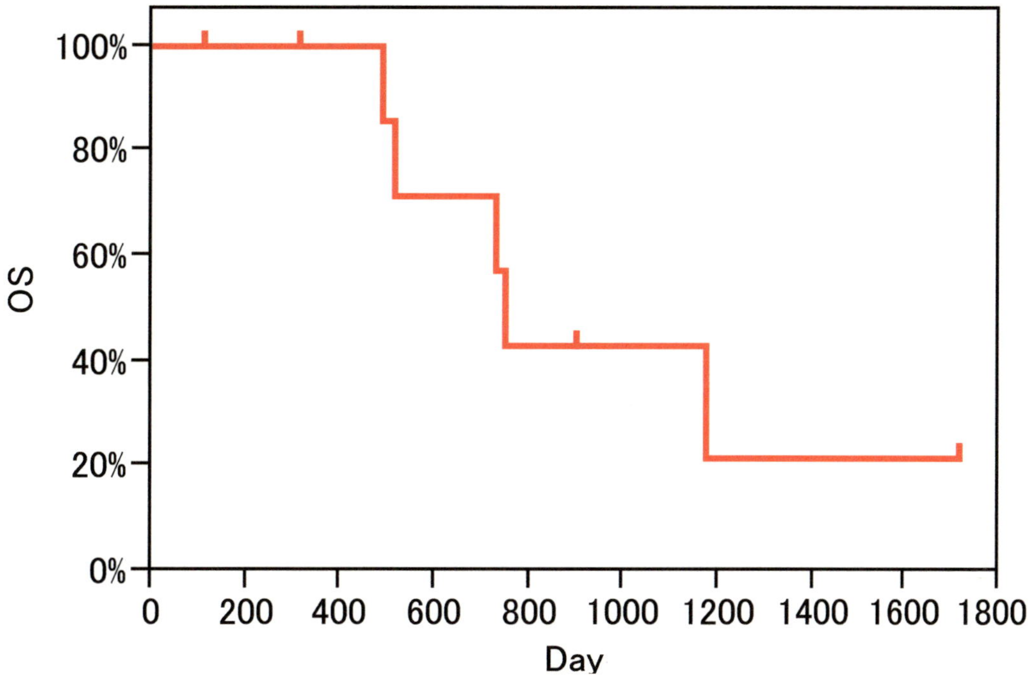

Fig. 3. Overall survival (OS) in patients receiving PSC therapy
Kaplan-Meier analysis of OS in 10 patients showed OS to be 747 days (95% CI: 488–1714 days).

3.3 Adverse effects

Adverse effects during PSC triple therapy were assessed in all 10 patients (Table 3). The most frequently observed severe (grades 3 and 4) toxicity was neutropenia (6 cases, 60%). Febrile neutropenia was observed in only one case (10%). As for non-hematological toxicities, severe anorexia and mucositis (grade 3) were observed in one case. Neither renal dysfunction nor hand-foot syndrome occurred in this study. There were essentially no differences in toxicity between patients with versus without prior chemotherapy.

4. Discussion

A prospective study of PSC triple therapy was conducted for metastatic or recurrent gastric cancer in our hospital. There have been few studies on the use of these three agents in unresectable gastric cancer. Iwase, et al. recommended the following doses: paclitaxel 120 mg/m^2, cisplatin 60 mg/m^2, and S-1 70 mg/m^2, based on the multicenter phase II study (Iwase, et al, 2010). Our patients were treated according to this regimen. This triple combination therapy yielded a high clinical response rate (70%) and a very high disease control rate (100%). In Japan, S-1/ cisplatin should be regarded as a reference regimen. In terms of survival effects, PSC triple therapy (median OS: 747 days [95% CI, 488–1714 days]) was apparently superior to S-1/ cisplatin, for which OS ranged from 10.4 to 13.0 months (Koizumi, et al, 2008 ; Lenz, et al, 2007). PSC appears to be more beneficial than other triple

Toxicity (n = 10)	Grade		
	2	**3**	**4**
Hematological toxicity			
Leucopenia	5	3	1
Neutropenia	3	4	2
Thrombocytopenia	3	1	0
Anemia	4	2	0
Non-hematological toxicity			
Skin rash	1	0	0
Mucositis	0	1	0
Diarrhea	0	1	0
Anorexia	3	1	0
Nausea	1	1	0
Vomiting	1	0	0
Liver dysfunction	1	0	0

Table 3. Toxicity incidence
Grade is based on the National Cancer Institute common toxicity criteria, version 4.0.

combination therapies (OS; DCF therapy 9.2 months, DSC therapy 687 days) (Sato, et. al, 2010; van Custem, et al, 2006).

In this trial, all toxicities were manageable and no patients died due to adverse effects. Neutropenia was the most common toxicity, but febrile neutropenia occurred in only one patient, who also had severe mucositis and diarrhea during the same (5th) course of PSC therapy. Continuous infusion of cisplatin for 24 hours induces nausea and vomiting, but the toxicity was milder than that associated with bolus injection of cisplatin. In addition, since June, 2010 we have routinely used aprepitant (Warr, et. al, 2005) to prevent gastrointestinal symptoms induced by cisplatin. Aprepitant remarkably reduces both the incidence and degree of vomiting, nausea, and anorexia.

Our prospective study further support the results of a phase II study (Iwase, et al, 2010) indicating that triple combination chemotherapy consisting of paclitaxel, S-1, and cisplatin had a favorable safety profile with encouraging efficacy against inoperable advanced gastric cancer. This PSC regimen is the major candidates for becoming the standard treatment for advanced gastric cancer. The results of controlled studies comparing PSC triple therapy with S-1/ cisplatin therapy are eagerly anticipated.

5. References

Hohenberger P, Gretshel S. Gastric cancer. Lancet 362: 305-315, 2003.

Shirasaka T, Shimamoto Y, Ohshino H, et al. Development of a novel form of an oral 5-fluorouracil derivative (S1) directed to the potentiation of the tumor selective cytotoxicity of 5-5-fluorouracil by two biochemical modulations. Anticancer Drugs 7: 548-557, 1996.

Scanlon KJ, Newmann EM, Lu Y, et al. Biochemical basis for cisplatin and 5-fluorouracil synergism in human ovarian carcinoma cells. Proc Natl Acad Sci USA 83: 8923-8925, 1986.

Lenz HJ, Lee FC, Haller DG, et al. Extended safety and efficacy data on S-1 plus cisplatin in patients with untreated, advanced gastric carcinoma in a multicenter phase II study. Cancer 109: 33-40, 2007.

Koizumi W, Narahara H, Hara T, et al. S-1 plus cisplatin versus S-1 alone for first line treatment of advanced gastric cancer (SPIRITS trial): a phase III trial. Lancet Oncol 9: 215-221, 2008.

Iwase H, Shimada M, Tsuzuki T, et al. A phase II multicentric trial of S-1 combined with 24 h-infusion of cisplatin in patients with advanced gastric cancer. Anticancer Res 25: 1297-1302, 2005.

Ohtsu A, Boku N, Mochizuki Y, et al. An early phase II study of a 3-hour infusion of paclitaxel for advanced gastric cancer. Am J Clin Oncol 21: 416-419, 1998.

Sulkes A, Smyth J, Sessa C, et al. Docetaxel (Taxotere) in advanced gastric cancer: results of a Phase II clinical trial. EORTIC Early Clinical Trials Group. Br J Cancer 70: 380-383, 1994.

Yamaguchi K, Shimamura T, Hyodo I, et al. Phase I/ II study of docetaxel and S-1 in patients with advanced gastric cancer. Br J Cancer 94: 1803-1808, 2006.

Nakayama N, Koizumi W, Sasaki T, et al. A multicenter, phase I dose - escalating study of docetaxel, cisplatin and S-1 for advanced gastric cancer. Oncology 75: 1-7, 2008.

Sato Y, Takayama T, Sagawa T, et al. Phase II study of S-1, docetaxel, and cisplatin combination chemotherapy in patients with unresectable metastatic gastric cancer. Cancer Chemother Pharmacol 66: 721-728, 2010.

Kang HJ, Chang HM, Kim TW, et al. A phase II study of paclitaxel and capecitabine as a first-line combination chemotherapy for advanced gastric cancer. Br J Cancer 98: 316-322, 2008.

Ina K, Kataoka T, Takeuchi Y, et al. Pathological complete response induced by the combination therapy of S-1 and 24-h infusion of cisplatin in two cases initially diagnosed as inoperable advanced gastric cancer. Oncology Reports 20: 259-264, 2008.

Japanese Research Society for Gastric Cancer: Japanese Classification of Gastric Carcinoma. Tokyo, Japan, Kanehara, 1995.

Iwase H, Ina K, Goto H, et al. Extended safety and efficacy data on triple combination therapy using S-1, cisplatin, and paclitaxel in patients with advanced gastric cancer in a multicenter phase II study. ASCO 28: 15, 2010.

Van Custem E, Moiseyenko VM, Tjulandin S, et al. Phase III study of docetaxel and cisplatin plus fluorouracil compared with cisplatin and fluorouracil as first-line therapy for advanced gastric cancer: a report of the V325 Study Group. J Clin Oncol 24 : 4991-4997, 2006.

Warr DG, Hesketh PJ, Gralla RJ, et al. Efficacy and tolerability of aprepitant for the prevention of chemotherapy-induced nausea and vomiting in patients with breast cancer after moderately emetogenic chemothrapy. J Clin Oncol 23 : 2822-2830, 2005.

Part 4

A Rare Gastric Carcinoma

8

A Rare Gastric Carcinoma - Neuroendocrine Tumors

Petar Svorcan, Jelena Djordjevic and Branko Maksimovic
Zvezdara Medical Center
Belgrade,
Serbia

1. Introduction

Neuroendocrine tumors, or more properly gastro-entero-pancreatic tumors (GEP-NETs), are cancers of the interface between the endocrine (hormonal) system and the nervous system. A neuroendocrine tumor begins in the hormone-producing cells of the body's neuroendocrine system, which is made up of cells that are a cross between traditional endocrine cells (or hormone-producing cells) and nerve cells. Neuroendocrine cells are found throughout the body in organs, such as the lungs and gastrointestinal tract (such as the stomach and intestines), and perform specific functions, such as regulating the air and blood flow through the lungs and controlling the speed at which food is moved through the gastrointestinal tract (1).

2. NETs epidemiology and characteristics

Neuroendocrine tumors (NETs) are rare, slow-growing neoplasms characterized by their ability to store and secrete different peptides and neuroamines. Some of these substances cause specific clinical syndromes, whereas other may have elevated plasma or urine levels that are not associated with specific syndromes or symptom complexes. The biochemical markers are those hormones or amines secreted by the neuroendocrine cells from which these tumors are derived. Some of these are not specific to any tumor, but are produced and secreted by most NETs, whereas other biochemical markers are more specific to the type of tumor and where their quantification can lead to the suspicion or confirmation of the presence of such a tumor (2). There are many types of neuroendocrine tumors, such as: pheochromocytoma, Merkel cell cancer, and neuroendocrine carcinoma, and also other types of cancer that begin in hormone-producing cells, including endocrine tumors, carcinoid tumors, thymoma, thyroid cancer, and islet cell tumors. Approximately 60% of neuroendocrine tumors are not able to be described as a specific type of cancer other than neuroendocrine carcinoma. Neuroendocrine carcinoma can be found in a number of places in the body, including the lungs, brain, and gastrointestinal tract. The annual incidence of NETs has risen to 40 to 50 cases per million, perhaps because of better diagnosis and the availability of highly specific and sensitive ways to measure these tumors products, improved immunohistochemistry, and enhanced techniques for tumor detection (3). There are a number of impediments to the diagnosis of these tumors. They are rare, comprising less than 2% of gastrointestinal (GI) malignancies, and are therefore not high on the list of causes of specific symptom complexes. Symptoms themselves are often nonspecific and do not lend themselves readily to identifying the specific underlying tumor. In addition, the manifestations are protean and mimic a variety of disorders. Tumors may be found incidentally on laparoscopy for abdominal pain or during the surgical removal of an appendix or even during a computerized tomographic scan of the abdomen for unexplained symptoms (3,4).

3. Classification of GEP-NETs by site of origin and by symptoms

The clinical behavior of NETs is extremely variable; they may be functioning or not functioning, ranging from very slow-growing tumors (well-differentiated NETs), which are the majority, to highly aggressive and very malignant tumors (poorly differentiated NETs) (5).

Classification	Biological behavior	Metastases	Ki-67 index (%)†	Histological differentiation	Infiltration/ angioinvasion	Tumor size (cm)
Well-differentiated NET	Benign	–‡; ±§	<2	Well	–	≤1
Well-differentiated neuroendocrine carcinoma	Low malignancy	±	>2	Well	+	>2‡; >3§
Poorly-differentiated neuroendocrine carcinoma	High malignancy	+	>30	Poor	+	Any size

†Identical to MIB1.
‡Gastrointestinal neuroendocrine tumor.
§Pancreatic neuroendocrine tumor.
NET: Neuroendocrine tumor.

Table 1. WHO classification of neuroendocrine tumors.

3.1 Nonfunctioning NETs

Nonfunctioning NETs are not associated with a distinct hormonal syndrome so are more difficult to detect than functioning NETs; owing to this, patients generally present late with large primary tumors and advanced disease. However, nonfunctioning NETs may secrete bioactive hormones or amines at subclinical levels, or secrete compounds that lead to other, still under-recognized hormonal syndromes. They can also cause nonspecific symptoms related to increased tumor mass and/or metastases such as weight loss, bleeding or abdominal pain.

3.2 Functioning NETs

NETs can arise in different organs and from different cell types and so present a clinical challenge to physicians owing to their diversity and the variety of symptoms they cause.

Functioning NETs are characterized by the hormones they produce and/or the symptoms they cause; clinical symptoms are typically observed following metastasis to the liver.

3.3 GEP-NETs classification

The vast majority of GEP-NETs fall into two nearly distinct categories: carcinoids, and pancreatic endocrine tumors (PETs). Despite great behavioral differences between the two, they are grouped together as GEP-NETs because of similarities in cell structure. PETs (1-2% of all pancreatic tumors) may secrete hormones (as a result, perhaps, of impaired storage ability), and those hormones can wreak symptomatic havoc on the body. Those PETs that do not secrete hormones are called *nonfunctioning* tumors. Secretory (*functioning*) tumors are classified by the hormone most strongly secreted - for example, insulinoma, which produces excessive insulin, and gastrinoma, which produces excessive gastrin. Carcinoid tumors are further classified, depending on the point of origin, as foregut (lung, thymus, stomach, and duodenum) or midgut (distal ileum and proximal colon) or hindgut (distal colon and rectum). Less than one percent of carcinoid tumors originate in the pancreas. But for many tumors, the point of origin is unknown. Carcinoid tumors tend to grow much more slowly than PETs (2,6).

3.4 Carcinoid syndrome

A carcinoid tumor may produce serotonin (5-HT), a biogenic amine that causes a specific set of symptoms including

- flushing
- diarrhea or increase in number of bowel movements
- weight loss
- weight gain
- heart palpitations
- congestive heart failure (CHF)
- asthma
- acromegaly
- Cushing's syndrome

This set of symptoms is called *carcinoid syndrome* which occurs in approximately 10% of patients with metastatic NETs. It is characterized by flushing (63–94% of patients), diarrhea (68–84%), abdominal pain (10–55%), telangiectasia (25%) and bronchoconstriction (3–19%). Carcinoid crisis is the most immediate life-threatening complication of carcinoid syndrome and is thought to result from a massive release of bioactive products from the tumor. Crises can occur spontaneously, but often arise in response to stress, anesthesia, chemotherapy or surgery. Symptoms are an exacerbation of the usual clinical symptoms of carcinoid syndrome, including severe flushing with or without bronchospasm, tachycardia and hypo/hypertension. Failure to effectively manage carcinoid syndrome can lead to exposure of the heart to high levels of vasoactive substances released from hepatic metastases, which causes carcinoid heart disease; between 10–20% of patients with carcinoid syndrome have heart disease at diagnosis. Carcinoid heart disease is characterized by plaque-like, fibrous thickening of the endocardium (classically on the right side of the heart); tricuspid and pulmonary valves; right-sided carcinoid heart disease is associated with substantial morbidity and mortality (7-10).

3.5 Summary of GEP - NETs classification (2,11,12)

- carcinoids (about two thirds of GEP-NETs)
    - with carcinoid syndrome (about 10 percent of carcinoids)
    - without carcinoid syndrome (about 90 percent of carcinoids)
- PET s (about one third of GEP-NETs)
    - nonfunctioning (15 to 30 percent of PETs)
    - functioning (70 to 85 percent of PETs)
        - gastrinoma, producing excessive gastrin and causing Zollinger-Ellison Syndrome (ZES)
        - insulinoma, producing excessive insulin
        - glucagonoma, producing excessive glucagon
        - vasoactive intestinal peptideoma (VIPoma), producing excessive vasoactive intestinal peptide (VIP)
        - PPoma, producing excessive pancreatic polypeptide (often classed with nonfunctioning PETs)
        - somatostatinoma, producing excessive somatostatin
        - watery diarrhea, hypokalemia-achlorhydria (WDHA)
        - CRHoma, producing excessive corticotropin-releasing hormonse (CRH)
        - calcitoninoma, producing excessive calcitonin
        - GHRHoma, producing excessive growth-hormone-releasing hormone (GHRH)
        - neurotensinoma, producing excessive neurotensin
        - ACTHoma, producing excessive adrenocorticotropic hormone (ACTH)
        - GRFoma, producing excessive Growth hormone-releasing factor (GRF)
        - parathyroid hormone–related peptide tumor
- Other NETs
    - medullary carcinoma of the thyroid
    - Merkel cell cancer (trabecular cancer)
    - small-cell lung cancer (SCLC)
    - large-cell neuroendocrine carcinoma (of the lung)
    - extrapulmonary small cell carcinomas (ESCC or EPSCC)in general
    - neuroendocrine carcinoma of the cervix
    - Multiple Endocrine Neoplasia type 1 (MEN-1 or MEN1) (usually nonfunctioning) (also causing ZES)
    - Multiple Endocrine Neoplasia type 2 (MEN-2 or MEN2)
    - neurofibromatosis type 1
    - tuberous sclerosis
    - von Hippel-Lindau (VHL) disease
    - neuroblastoma
    - pheochromocytoma (phaeochromocytoma)
    - paraganglioma
    - neuroendocrine tumor of the anterior pituitary
    - Carney's complex

4. Metastases and malignancy

GEP-NETs are often malignant, since the primary site often eludes detection for years, sometimes decades – during which time the tumor has the opportunity to metastasize. The most common metastatic sites are the liver, the lymph nodes, and the bones. Liver metastases are so frequent and have such prominent blood supply that for many patients, they dominate the course of the cancer (13).

5. Well-differentiated neuroendocrine (carcinoid) tumors of the stomach

Neuroendocrine tumors (NETs) of the stomach comprise less than 1% of gastric neoplasms. In the pre-endoscopy era,they comprised 1.9% of all carcinoids, but in more recent studies, 10% to 30% of all carcinoids are reported in the stomach. They can be subclassified into 3 distinct groups: those associated with chronic atrophic gastritis/pernicious anemia (type 1; 70%-80%), those associated with Zollinger-Ellison syndrome (ZES) with multiple endocrine neoplasia type I (MEN I) (type 2; 5%), and sporadic NETs of the stomach (type 3; 15%-20%) (13-15).

5.1 Etiology

Both types 1 and 2 NETs of the stomach are associated with hypergastrinemia (Table 2). High levels of gastrin are thought to result in hyperplasia of the enterochromaffin-like cells in the stomach, ultimately leading to hyperplastic lesions and small, often multiple carcinoid tumors. In contrast to types 1 and 2 carcinoids, type 3 carcinoids develop in the absence of hypergastrinemia and tend to pursue an aggressive clinical course. Type 1 carcinoids are generally small and frequently multiple; limited to the mucosa-submucosa, and metastases occur in less than 2.5% to lymph nodes and less than 2.5%% to the liver. Type 2 carcinoids are almost always multiple and generally small (<1 cm) and are usually limited to the mucosa-submucosa, but are slightly more aggressive than type 1 carcinoids, with up to 30% showing lymph node metastases, and up to 10% may show liver metastases.Type 3 carcinoids are usually single, generally larger (>1 cm in 70%), and invasive through the submucosa and deeper in most cases (>75%); 70% had accompanying lymph node metastases, and 69% had distant metastases (16,17).

	Hypergastrinemia	Gastric acid Secretion	Typical Size, cm	No. tumors	Clinical Features
Type 1 (in setting of chronic atrophic gastritis type A)	Yes (as a result of achlorhydria)	Low	< 1	Multifocal	Rarely invasive; endoscopic removal often adequate
Type 2 (in setting of ZES)	Yes (as a result of ectopic gastrin secretion)	High	< 1	Multifocal	Rarely invasive; may respond to somatostatin analogs
Type 3 (sporadic)	No	Normal	> 1	Solitary	Frequently invasive and metastatic

Table 2. Types of gastric NETs

5.2 Pathological classification

In general, NETs of the stomach and other NETs are divided into well-differentiated and poorly differentiated categories. The concept of differentiation is linked to the grade of the tumors (see below), but there are subtle differences between differentiation and grade. Differentiation refers to the extent to which the neoplastic cells resemble their nonneoplastic counterparts. In NETs, well-differentiated examples have characteristic "organoid" arrangements of the tumor cells, with nesting, trabecular, or gyriform patterns. The cells are relatively uniform and produce abundant neurosecretory granules, reflected in the strong and diffuse immunoexpression of neuroendocrine markers such as chromogranin A (CGA) and synaptophysin. Poorly differentiated NETs less closely resemble nonneoplastic neuroendocrine cells and have a more sheet-like or diffuse architecture, irregular nuclei, and less cytoplasmic granularity. Immunoexpression of neuroendocrine markers is usually more limited. Grade, on the other hand, refers to the inherent biologic aggressiveness of the tumor. Low-grade NETs are relatively indolent, high-grade tumors are extremely aggressive, and intermediate-grade examples have a less predictable, moderately aggressive course. In general, well-differentiated NETs are either low or intermediate grade, and poorly differentiated NETs are considered high grade in all cases (Table 3) (18-22).

Differentiation	Grade
Well differentiated	Low grade (ENETS G1) Intermediate grade (ENETS G2)
Poorly differentiated	High grade (ENETS G3)

Table 3. Differentiation of gastric NETs

<table>
<tr><th>Grade</th><th>Lung, Thymus (WHO)</th><th>GEP NETs (ENETS)</th><th>GEP NETs (WHO 2010)</th></tr>
<tr><td>Low grade</td><td>Carcinoid tumor</td><td>NET grade 1 (G1)</td><td>Neuroendocrine neoplasm grade 1</td></tr>
<tr><td>Intermediate grade</td><td>Atypical carcinoid tumor</td><td>NET grade 2 (G2)</td><td>Neuroendocrine neoplasm grade 2</td></tr>
<tr><td rowspan="2">High grade</td><td>Small cell carcinoma</td><td>Neuroendocrine carcinoma grade 3 (G3), small cell carcinoma</td><td>Neuroendocrine carcinoma grade 3, small cell carcinoma</td></tr>
<tr><td>Large cell neuroendocrine carcinoma</td><td>Neuroendocrine carcinoma grade 3 (G3), large cell neuroendocrine</td><td>Neuroendocrine carcinoma grade 3, large cell neuroendocrine carcinoma</td></tr>
<tr><td colspan="4">The grade of the tumor must be included in the pathology report, along with a reference to the specific grading system being used. Unqualified terms such as neuroendocrine tumor or neuroendocrine carcinoma without reference to grade do not provide adequate pathology information.</td></tr>
</table>

Table 4. Differentiation of gastric Nets (2)

Table 4 displays a comparison of the various systems of nomenclature currently in use for NETs, along with for which organ systems each system is most commonly used.
Figures 1-3 are presenting histology evaluation of neuroendocrine gastric carcinoma-large cell type, that demonstrates trabecula and islet of round cells with rare eosinophilic cytoplasm. The nuclei are atypical, hyperchromatic, moderately pleomorphic, without prominent nucleolus. The stroma is edematous. Vascular invasion in mucosa and submucosa is also detected (Stained H&E - Figure 1). Cytological immunophenotypes includes: marked and diffuse immunoreactivity in the majority of the cells to neuron specific-enolase (NSE) - (Figure 2), chromogranin A(Figure 3) and synaptophysin.

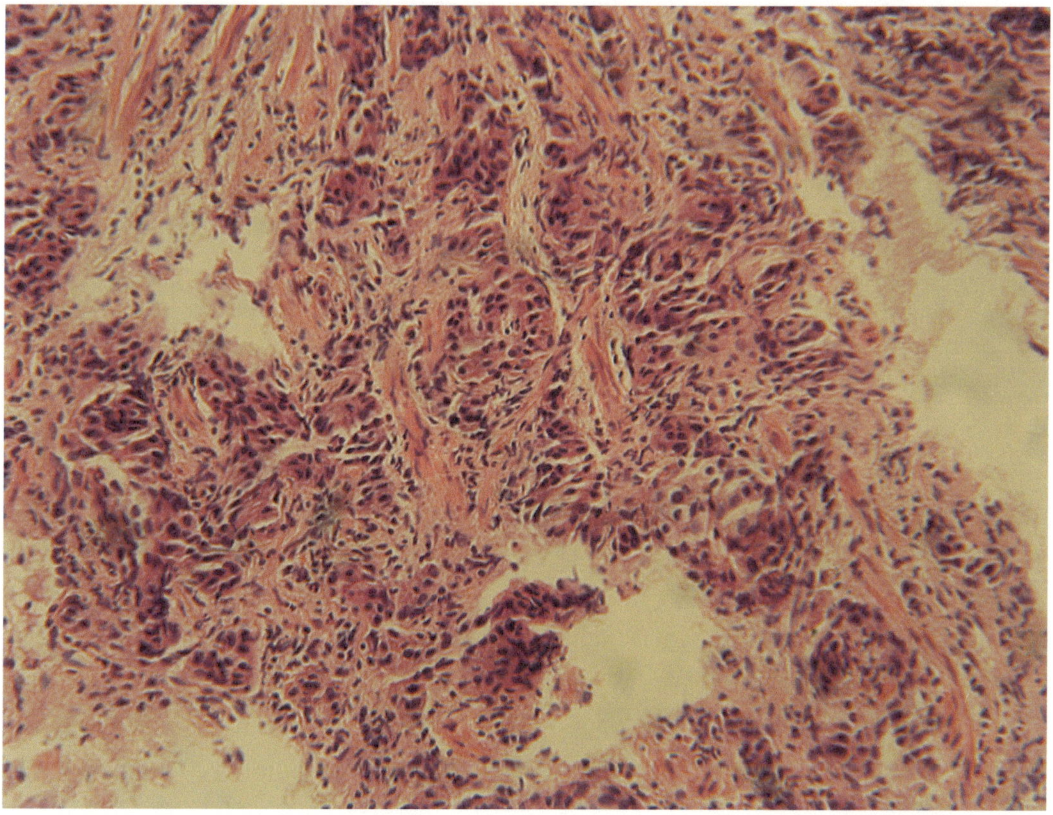

Fig. 1. Neuroendocrine gastric carcinoma-large cell type, Stained H&E, x400. Courtesy by Prof S.Usaj

The American Joint Committee on Cancer (AJCC) has recently published a new TNM staging manual that includes NETs of all anatomical sites, and the ENETS has previously published recommendations for TNM staging of GEP NETs. dditionally, the staging criteria for both systems rely predominantly on the size of the tumor and the extent of invasion into similar landmarks as used for the staging of nonneuroendocrine carcinomas of the same sites. It is recommended that the extent of involvement of these structures be specifically indicated in the pathology reports, in addition to providing a TNM stage based on a system that is specifically referenced (Table 5) (23-26). Figures 4 and 5 represent T2 and M1 GEP NET thru the EUS image.

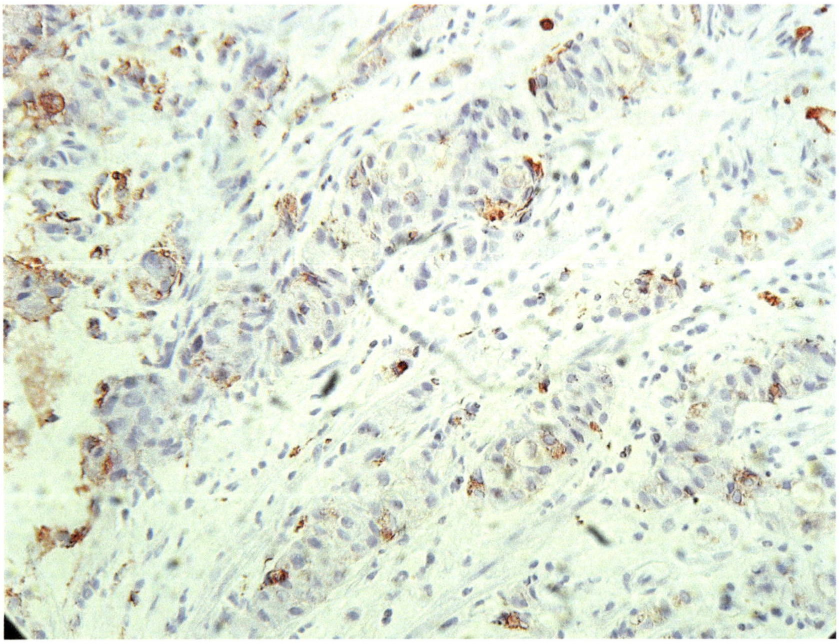

Fig. 2. Neuroendocrine tumor cells of the stomach wall -Immunostaining - NSE (LSAB+ , x200). Courtesy by Prof S.Usaj

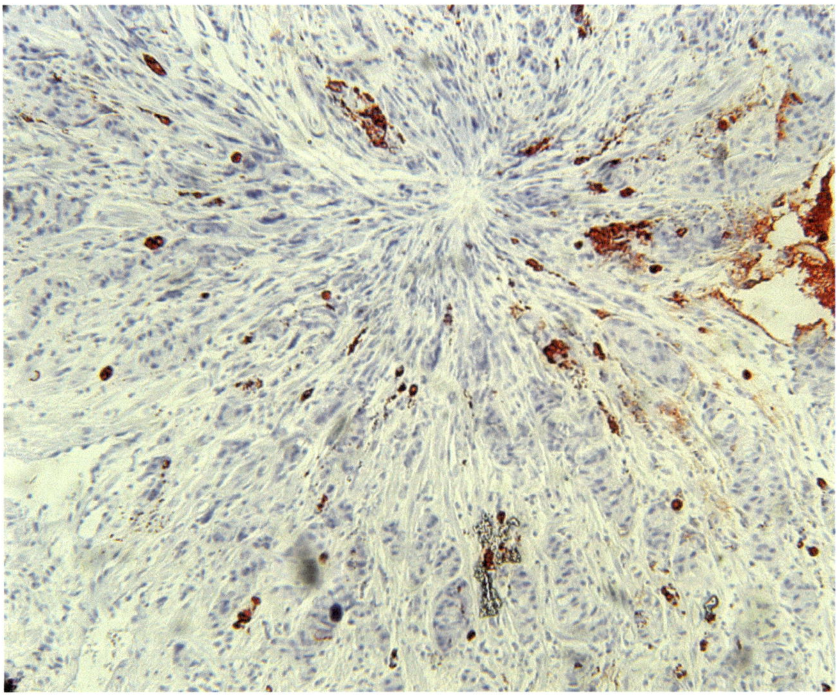

Fig. 3. Neuroendocrine tumor cells of the stomach wall- Immunostaining - chromogranin A (LSAB+ , x200). Courtesy by Prof S.Usaj

<table>
<tr><th colspan="4">AJCC
Primary tumor (T)</th><th colspan="4">ENETS
T-Primary Tumor</th></tr>
<tr><td colspan="2">TX</td><td colspan="2">Primary tumor cannot be assessed</td><td colspan="2">TX</td><td colspan="2">Primary tumor cannot be assessed</td></tr>
<tr><td colspan="2">T0</td><td colspan="2">No evidence of primary tumor</td><td colspan="2">T0</td><td colspan="2">No evidence of primary tumor</td></tr>
<tr><td colspan="2">Tis</td><td colspan="2">Carcinoma in situ/dysplasia (tumor size <0.5mm), confined to mucosa</td><td colspan="2">—</td><td colspan="2"></td></tr>
<tr><td colspan="2">T1</td><td colspan="2">Tumor invades lamina propria or submucosa and ≤ 1 cm</td><td colspan="2">T1</td><td colspan="2">Tumor invades lamina propria or submucosa and ≤ 1 cm</td></tr>
<tr><td colspan="2">T2</td><td colspan="2">Tumor invades muscularis propria or > 1 cm</td><td colspan="2">T2</td><td colspan="2">Tumor invades muscularis propria or > 1 cm</td></tr>
<tr><td colspan="2">T3</td><td colspan="2">Tumor penetrates subserosa</td><td colspan="2">T3</td><td colspan="2">Tumor invades pancreas or retroperitoneum</td></tr>
<tr><td colspan="2">T4</td><td colspan="2">Tumor invades serosa (visceral peritoneum) or other organs or adjacent structures</td><td colspan="2">T4</td><td colspan="2">Tumor invades peritoneum or other organs</td></tr>
<tr><td colspan="2">Regional Lymph nodes (N)</td><td colspan="2"></td><td colspan="2">N-Regional Lymph Nodes</td><td colspan="2"></td></tr>
<tr><td colspan="2">NX</td><td colspan="2">Regional lymph node(s) cannot be assessed</td><td colspan="2">NX</td><td colspan="2">Regional lymph node(s) cannot be assessed</td></tr>
<tr><td colspan="2">N0</td><td colspan="2">No regional lymph node metastasis</td><td colspan="2">N0</td><td colspan="2">No regional lymph node metastasis</td></tr>
<tr><td colspan="2">N1</td><td colspan="2">Regional lymph node metastasis</td><td colspan="2">N1</td><td colspan="2">Regional lymph node metastasis</td></tr>
<tr><td colspan="2">Distant metastasis (M)</td><td colspan="2"></td><td colspan="2">M-distant metastasis</td><td colspan="2"></td></tr>
<tr><td colspan="2">—</td><td colspan="2"></td><td colspan="2">MX</td><td colspan="2">Distant metastasis cannot be assessed</td></tr>
<tr><td colspan="2">M0</td><td colspan="2">No distant metastasis</td><td colspan="2">M0</td><td colspan="2">No distant metastasis</td></tr>
<tr><td colspan="2">M1</td><td colspan="2">Distant metastasis</td><td colspan="2">M1</td><td colspan="2">Distant metastasis</td></tr>
<tr><td>Stage</td><td>T</td><td>N</td><td>M</td><td>Stage</td><td>T</td><td>N</td><td>M</td></tr>
<tr><td>0</td><td>Tis</td><td>N0</td><td>M0</td><td>0</td><td>Tis</td><td>N0</td><td>M0</td></tr>
<tr><td>I</td><td>T1</td><td>N0</td><td>M0</td><td>I</td><td>T1</td><td>N0</td><td>M0</td></tr>
<tr><td>IIA</td><td>T2</td><td>N0</td><td>M0</td><td>IIa</td><td>T2</td><td>N0</td><td>M0</td></tr>
<tr><td>IIB</td><td>T3</td><td>N0</td><td>M0</td><td>IIb</td><td>T3</td><td>N0</td><td>M0</td></tr>
<tr><td>IIIA</td><td>T4</td><td>N0</td><td>M0</td><td>IIIa</td><td>T4</td><td>N0</td><td>M0</td></tr>
<tr><td>IIIB</td><td>Any T</td><td>N1</td><td>M0</td><td>IIIb</td><td>Any T</td><td>N1</td><td>M0</td></tr>
<tr><td>IV</td><td>Any T</td><td>Any N</td><td>M1</td><td>IV</td><td>Any T</td><td>Any N</td><td>M1</td></tr>
</table>

Table 5. The TNM NETs classification

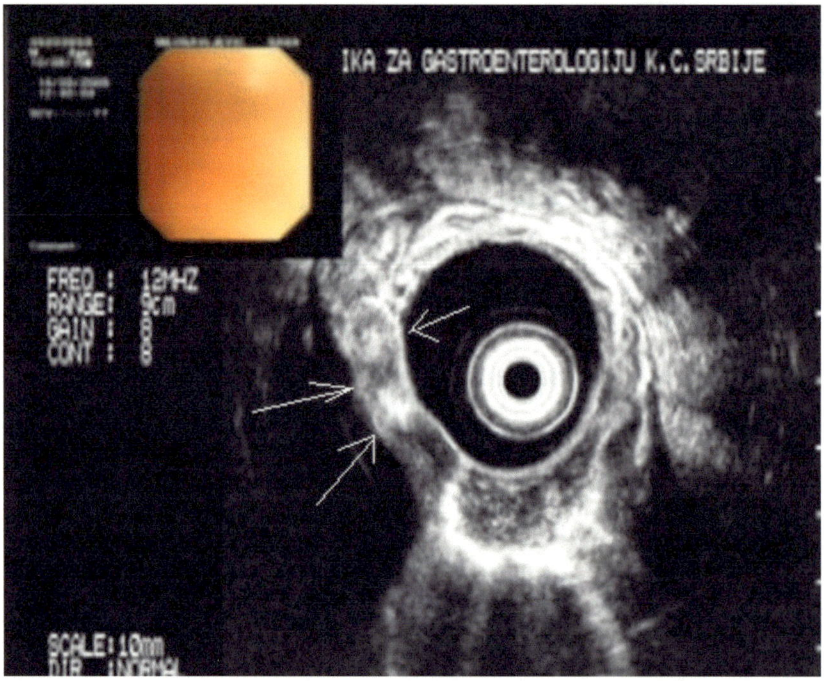

Fig. 4. EUS image: T2 tumor of the stomach wall. Courtesy by Prof M.Krstic

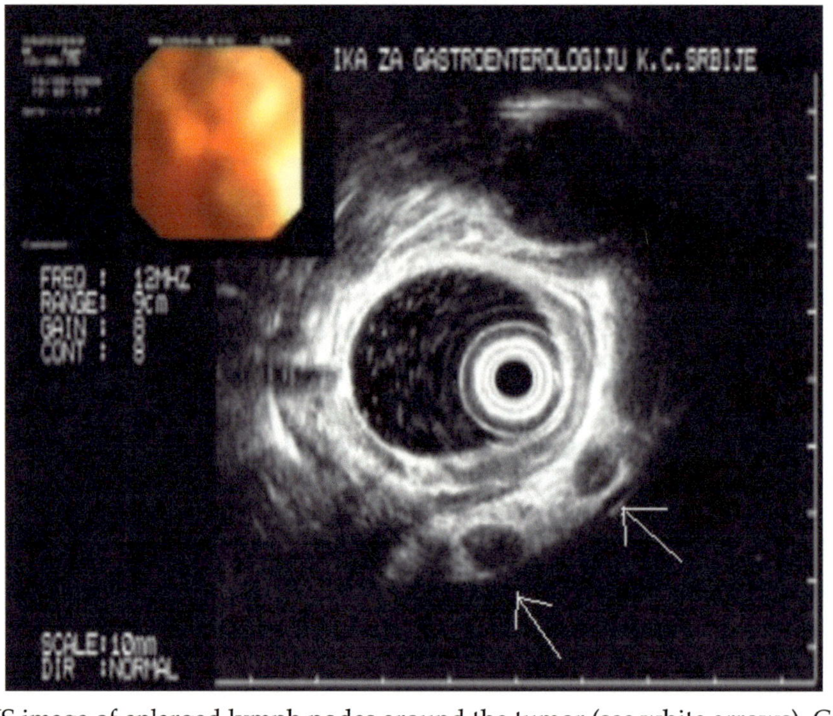

Fig. 5. EUS image of enlarged lymph nodes around the tumor (see white arrows). Courtesy by Prof M.Krstic

6. Imaging

Most NETs of the stomach are directly imaged and diagnosed during endoscopy. For larger lesions, endoscopic ultrasound (EUS) may be performed to assess whether the NETs of the stomach is invasive. Cross-sectional imaging with computed tomography (CT) or magnetic resonance imaging (MRI) is recommended to assess for metastases in patients with type 1 or 2 NETs of the stomach more than 2 cm in diameter, or for patients with type 3 NETs of the stomach in whom metastatic risk is a concern. Neuroendocrine tumors are generally vascular tumors that enhance intensely with intravenous contrast during early arterial phases of imaging with washout during the delayed portal venous phase. The key to detecting small NETs on CT is to maximize the contrast between the tumor and the adjacent normal parenchyma. For abdominal and pelvic imaging, recommendation is multiphasic CT that includes the arterial phase and the portal venous phase. Rapid intravenous bolus of intravenous contrast is also recommended. Thin sectioning and the use of a negative oral contrast agent also may be helpful in detecting small primary tumor in the small bowel that may not otherwise be seen. Magnetic resonance imaging is preferred over CT for patients with a history of allergy to iodine contrast material or for those with renal insufficiency. Somatostatin receptor scintigraphy (SRS) provides a second useful imaging modality for the detection of metastatic disease in patients with malignant NETs of the stomach. Indium In 111-labeled somatostatin analog [^{111}In-DTPA^{0}]octreotide was developed for scintigraphy of NETs. It shares the receptor-binding profile of octreotide, which makes it a good radiopharmaceutical for imaging of somatostatin receptor 2- and receptor 5-positive tumors. The overall sensitivity of [^{111}In-DTPA^{0}]octreotide scintigraphy seems to be about 80% to 90%. Unlike cross-sectional imaging, which is generally site directed, [^{111}In-DTPA^{0}]octreotide scintigraphy is done as whole-body imaging and thus can detect disease at unsuspected sites. Chest x-ray can be used as a screening examination for patients without evidence of thoracic disease (27,29).

7. Biochemical monitoring

Fasting serum gastrin levels are important to differentiate types 1 and 2 NETs of the stomach from type 3. 5-Hydroxyindoleacetic acid (5-HIAA) levels are generally not useful in patients with NETs of the stomach, because development of the carcinoid syndrome is uncommon. Furthermore, carcinoid syndrome, if it occurs in these patients, is reported to be characteristically atypical with normal serotonin and 5-HIAA levels, although a recent study reports the typical carcinoid syndrome can occur in rare patients with NETs of the stomach. Plasma CGA levels are recommended because CGA is frequently elevated in both patients with types 1 and 2 as well as type 3 NETs of the stomach, and changes in CGA levels may be helpful in the follow-up. Chromogranin A should be used with caution as a marker of disease activity in patients treated with somatostatin analogs, because these agents significantly reduce plasma CGA levels, a change that may be more reflective of changes in hormonal synthesis and release from tumor cells than an actual reduction in tumor mass. In patients on stable doses of somatostatin analogs, consistent increases in plasma CGA levels over time may reflect loss of secretory control and/or tumor growth. Plasma CGA levels have also been shown to have a prognostic value in patients with metastatic disease (16,17,30,31).

8. Management of localized NETs of the stomach

Because types 1 and 2 NETs of the stomach generally pursue an indolent course, tumors less than 2 cm (up to 6) should be resected endoscopically, with subsequent interval follow-up (15,27,32). Patients with tumors measuring more than 2 cm, with recurrent tumors or with more than 6 polyps, generally require more aggressive management, and local surgical resection is recommended. In patients with type 1 NETs of the stomach arising in the setting of chronic atrophic gastritis, antrectomy may be performed to eliminate the source of gastric production. Antrectomy has been reported to result in tumor regression in such cases. In patients with type 2 NETs of the stomach secondary to ZES/MEN I syndrome, treatment with somatostatin analogs may be initiated and has resulted in tumor regression.(33-35) The surgical management of type 3 isolated sporadic NETs of the stomach requires more aggressive surgery, generally with partial gastrectomy and lymph node dissection (Table 6). Surgery is the only therapy that can cure GEP-NETs. However, the typical delay in diagnosis, giving the tumor the opportunity to metastasize, makes most GEP-NETs ineligible for surgery (non-resectable). The most common nonsurgical therapy for all GEP-NETs is chemotherapy, although chemotherapy is reported to be largely ineffective for carcinoids, not particularly durable (long-lasting) for PETs, and inappropriate for PETs of nonpancreatic origin. When chemotherapy fails, the most common therapy, in the United States, is more chemotherapy, with a different set of agents. Some studies have shown that the benefit from one agent is not highly predictive of the benefit from another agent, except that the long-term benefit of any agent is likely to be low. Strong uptake of somatostatin analogs is a negative indication for chemo. There are two major somatostatin-analog-based targeted therapies. The first of the two therapies provides symptomatic relief for patients with secretory tumors. In effect, somatostatin given subcutaneously or intramuscularly

	Size, cm	No. tumors	Therapy	Clinical Features
Type 1 (in setting of chronic atrophic gastritis type A)	< 2	< 6	Resected endoscopically	Rarely invasive; endoscopic removal often adequate
	> 2	> 6	Local surgical resection/antrectomy	
Type 2 (in setting of ZES)	< 2	< 6	Resected endoscopically	Rarely invasive; may respond to somatostatin analogs
	> 2	> 6	Local surgical resection/antrectomy	
Type 3 (sporadic)	> 1	Solitary	Partial gastrectomy and lymph nodes resection	Frequently invasive and metastatic-Chemotherapy, chemotherapy with different agents

Table 6. Management of localized NETs of the stomach

"clogs up" the receptors, blocking the secretion of hormones from the tumor cells. The second of the two major somatostatin-analog-based targeted therapies is called *peptide receptor radionuclide therapy* (PRRT), though we might simply call it *hormone-delivered radiotherapy*. In this form of *radioisotope therapy* (RIT), radioactive substances (called *radionuclides* or *radioligands*) are chemically *conjugated* with hormones (peptides or neuroamines); the combination is given intravenously to a patient who has good uptake of the chosen hormone. The radioactive labelled hormones enter the tumor cells, and the attached radiation damages the tumor- and nearby cells. Not all cells are immediately killed this way. The process of tumor cells dying as result of this therapy can go on for several months, even up to two years. In patients with strongly overexpressing tumor cells, nearly all the radiation either gets into the tumors or is excreted in urine (10).

9. Management of metastatic NETs of the stomach

In general, metastatic NETs of the stomach, which are infrequent and therefore usually included in general studies including other more frequent malignant carcinoids (especially midgut), are treated in a similar fashion as these other malignant carcinoids. It has been proposed for the occasional, younger patient without any of these risk factors with a metastatic carcinoid tumor that is unresectable and limited to the liver that liver transplantation remains an option that should be considered (Table 7).

10. Hepatic resection and transplantation

A small percentage of patients (5%-15%) with metastatic liver disease with a limited number of hepatic metastases localized preferable to one lobe may be successfully treated with hepatic resection, providing both long-term symptomatic relief and likely increasing survival times. The number of patients with liver-isolated metastatic NETs in whom orthotopic liver transplantation (OLT) has been attempted remains small, resulting in the role of OLT in such patients being controversial and cannot, at this time, be routinely recommended (36-38).

11. Hepatic artery embolization

Hepatic arterial embolization is recommended as a palliative option in patients with hepatic metastases who are not candidates for surgical resection, have an otherwise preserved performance status, have disease primarily confined to the liver, and have a patent portal vein. The response rates associated with embolization, as measured either by decrease in hormonal secretion or by radiographic regression, are generally greater than 50% (39-41).

12. Cytotoxic chemotherapy

Because of its rarity, there have not been any specific studies of cytotoxic agents in only patients with malignant NETs of the stomach. However, with malignant carcinoids in general, cytotoxic chemotherapy plays only a limited role, and therefore, it is probable that similar results can be expected with malignant NETs of the stomach. Studies of single-agent therapy with 5-fluorouracil, streptozocin, or doxorubicin in patients with metastatic carcinoid tumors have shown that these agents are associated with only modest response rates (41,42).

13. Systemic treatment of metastatic disease

Patients with metastatic NETs of the stomach may develop an "atypical" carcinoid syndrome related to release of histamine and/or 5-HTP or rarely a typical carcinoid syndrome as seen in patients with metastatic midgut carcinoids. These patients frequently benefit from treatment with somatostatin analogs for symptom control. The addition of α-interferon to therapy with somatostatin analogs has been reported to be effective in controlling symptoms in patients with carcinoid syndrome who may be resistant to somatostatin analogs alone. Treatment with α-interferon may therefore be considered in patients with metastatic NETs of the stomach refractory to somatostatin analogs. In clinical trials, doses of α-interferon have ranged from 3 to 9 MU subcutaneously, administered from 3 to 7 times per week. The direct antineoplastic effects of somatostatin analogs either with or without interferon remain uncertain, although recent studies suggest they have a cytostatic effect in 40% to 70% of patients (41,42).

Metastasis or non resectable GEP NETs	Hepatic resection and transplantation
	Hepatic Artery Embolization
	Cytotoxic Chemotherapy
	Systemic treatment of metastatic disease- somatostatin analogs, interferon
	Radiofrequency Ablation and Cryoablation

Table 7. Management of metastatic NETs of the stomach

14. Radiofrequency ablation and cryoablation

Other approaches to the treatment of hepatic metastases include the use of radiofrequency ablation (RFA) and cryoablation, either alone or in conjunction with surgical debulking. These approaches can be performed using a percutaneous or laparoscopic approach.

15. Summary and conclusions

To conclude, neuroendocrine tumors are small, slow-growing neoplasms, usually with episodic expression that makes diagnosis difficult, erroneous, and often late; for these reasons, a high index of suspicion is needed, and it is important to understand the pathophysiology of each tumor to decide which biochemical markers are more useful and when they should be used. It is the purpose of this text to show the importance of recognizing, as early as possible, the clinical syndromes that suggest a NET as one of the differential diagnoses, and once suspected, look for the appropriate biochemical markers and radiological or other means that will confirm the diagnosis or confidently discard it. Ultimately, all 3 modalities are important to create a platform for monitoring response to therapy, determining prognosis, and choosing the right therapeutic intervention (43).

16. References

[1] Arnold R, Göke R, Wied M, Behr T. "Chapter 15 Neuroendocrine Gastro-Entero-Pancreatic (GEP) Tumors". In Scheppach W, Bresalier RS, Tytgat GNJ. *Gastrointestinal and Liver Tumors.* Berlin: Springer. pp. 2003; 195–233.

[2] Arnold R, Rinke A, Schmidt C, et al. Endocrine tumours of the gastrointestinal tract: chemotherapy. *Best Pract Res Clin Gastroenterol.* 2005; 19:649-656.

[3] Capella C, Solcia E, LH LS, et al. Endocrine tumours of the stomach. In: Hamilton SR, Aaltonen LA, eds. *Pathology and Genetics of Tumours of the Digestive System.* Lyon, France: IARC Press; 2000; 137-139.

[4] Delle Fave G, Capurso G, Milione M, et al. Endocrine tumours of the stomach. *Best Pract Res Clin Gastroenterol.* 2005; 19:659-673.

[5] Eckhauser F, Lloyd R, Thompson N, et al. Antrectomy for multicentric, argyrophil gastric carcinoids:a preliminary report. *Surgery.* 1988; 104:1046-1053.

[6] Fahy B, Tang L, Klimstra D, et al. Carcinoid of the rectum risk stratification (CaRRS): a strategy for preoperative outcome assessment. *Ann Surg Oncol.* 2007; 14:396-404

[7] Falconi M, Plockinger U, Kwekkeboom DJ, et al. Well-differentiated pancreatic non functioning tumors/carcinoma. *Neuroendocrinology.* 2006; 84:196-211.

[8] Gibril F, Reynolds JC, Lubensky IA, et al. Ability of somatostatin receptor scintigraphy to identify patients with gastric carcinoids: a prospective study. *J Nucl Med.* 2000; 41:1646-1656.

[9] Gupta S, Yao JC, Ahrar K, et al. Hepatic artery embolization and chemoembolization for treatment of patients with metastatic carcinoid tumors: the M.D. Anderson experience. *Cancer J.* 2003; 9:261-267.

[10] Hirschowitz BI, Griffith J, Pellegrin D, et al. Rapid regression of enterochromaffinlike cell gastric carcinoids in pernicious anemia after antrectomy. *Gastroenterology*. 1992; 102:1409-1418.

[11] Hochwald S, Zee S, Conlon K, et al. Prognostic factors in pancreatic endocrine neoplasms: an analysis of 136 cases with a proposal for low-grade and intermediate-grade groups. *J Clin Oncol*. 2002; 20:2633-2642.

[12] Hou W, Schubert ML. Treatment of gastric carcinoids. *Curr Treat Options Gastroenterol*. 2007; 10:123-133.

[13] Janson E, Holmberg L, Stridsberg M, et al. Carcinoid tumors: analysis of prognostic factors and survival in 301 patients from a referral center. *Ann Oncol*. 1997; 8:685-690.

[14] Kaltsas GA, Besser GM, Grossman AB. The diagnosis and medical management of advanced neuroendocrine tumors. *Endocr Rev*. 2004; 25:458-511.

[15] Kimura W, Kuroda A, Morioka YClinical pathology of endocrine tumors of the pancreas. Analysis of autopsy cases", *Dig Dis Sci*. 1991;36 (7): 933–42.

[16] Klöppel G, Perren A, Heitz PU.The gastroenteropancreatic neuroendocrine cell system and its tumors: the WHO classification. *Ann N Y Acad Sci*. 2004; 1014 (1): 13–27.

[17] Krenning EP, Kooij PPM, Bakker WH, et al. Radiotherapy with a radiolabeled somatostatin analogue, [^{111}In-DTPA-D-Phe1]-octreotide. *Ann N Y Acad Sci*. 1994; 733:496-506.

[18] Kvols LK. Carcinoid Tumors and the Carcinoid Syndrome: What's New in the Therapeutic Pipeline. *The Carcinoid Cancer Foundation: Carcinoid Symposium 2002*, http://www.carcinoid.org/pcf/lectures/docs/KVOLS.htm.

[19] Le Treut YP, Gregoire E, Belghiti J, et al. Predictors of long-term survival after liver transplantation for metastatic endocrine tumors: an 85-case French multicentric report. *Am J Transplant*. 2008; 8:1205-1213.

[20] Lin O, Olgac S, Green O, et al. Immunohistochemical staining of cytologic smears with MIB-1 helps distinguish low-grade from high-grade neuroendocrine neoplasms. *Am J Clin Pathol*. 2003;120:209-216.

[21] Massironi S, Sciola V, Peracchi M, et al. Neuroendocrine tumors of the gastro-entero-pancreatic system. *World J Gastroenterol*. 2008;14:5377-5384.

[22] Metz DC, Jensen RT. Gastrointestinal neuroendocrine tumors: pancreatic endocrine tumors. *Gastroenterology*. 2008; 135:1469-1492.

[23] Modlin IM, Lye KD, Kidd M. A 5-decade analysis of 13,715 carcinoid tumors. *Cancer*. 2003;97:934- 959.

[24] Modlin IM, Shapiro MD, Kidd M. Siegfried Oberndorfer: origins and perspectives of carcinoid tumors. *Hum Pathol*. 2004; 35 (12): 1440–51.

[25] Norton JA, Melcher ML, Gibril F, et al. Gastric carcinoid tumors in multiple endocrine neoplasia-1 patients with Zollinger-Ellison syndrome can be symptomatic, demonstrate aggressive growth, and require surgical treatment. *Surgery*. 2004;136:1267-1274.

[26] Olausson M, Friman S, Herlenius G, et al. Orthotopic liver or multivisceral transplantation as treatment of metastatic neuroendocrine tumors. *Liver Transpl.* 2007; 13:327-333.
[27] O'Toole D, Ruszniewski P. Chemoembolization and other ablative therapies for liver metastases of gastrointestinal endocrine tumours. *Best Pract Res Clin Gastroenterol.* 2005;, 19:585-594.
[28] Öberg K. Carcinoid Tumors: Current Concepts in Diagnosis and Treatment."*Oncologist* 3. 1998; (5): 339–345.
[29] Öberg K. Neuroendocrine Gastroenteropancreatic Tumours: Current Views on Diagnosis and Treatment. *Business Briefing: European Oncology Review 2005* ;90-2.
[30] Öberg K, Kvol L, Caplin M. Consensus report on the use of somatostatin analogs for the management of neuroendocrine tumors of the gastroenteropancreatic system. *Ann Oncol.* 2004; 15:966-973.
[31] Pascher A, Klupp J, Neuhaus P. Endocrine tumours of the gastrointestinal tract. Transplantation in the management of metastatic endocrine tumours. *Best Pract Res Clin Gastroenterol.* 2005; 19:637-648.
[32] Ramage JK, Davies AH, Ardill J, *et al.* "Guidelines for the management of gastroenteropancreatic neuroendocrine (including carcinoid) tumours, *Gut.* 2005; Suppl 4 (suppl_4): iv1–16.
[33] Rindi G, Bordi C, Rappel S, et al. Gastric carcinoids and neuroendocrine carcinomas: pathogenesis, pathology, and behavior. *World J Surg.* 1996; 20:168-172.
[34] Ruszniewski P, Delle Fave G, Cadiot G, et al. Well-differentiated gastric tumors/carcinomas. *Neuroendocrinology.* 2006; 84:158-164.
[35] Sarmiento JM, Que FG. Hepatic surgery for metastases from neuroendocrine tumors. *Surg Oncol Clin N Am.* 2003; 87:47-62.
[36] Sun W, Lipsitz S, Catalano P, et al. Phase II/III study of doxorubicin with fluorouracil compared with streptozocin with fluorouracil or dacarbazine in the treatment of advanced carcinoid tumors: Eastern Cooperative Oncology Group Study E1281. *J Clin Oncol.* 2005; 23;4897-4904.
[37] Tomassetti P, Migliori M, Caletti G, et al. Treatment of type II gastric carcinoid tumors with somatostatin analogs. *N Engl J Med.* 2000; 343:551-554.
[38] Toumpanakis C, Meyer T, Caplin ME. Cytotoxic treatment including embolization/chemoembolization for neuroendocrine tumours. *Best Pract Res Clin Endocrinol Metab.* 2007;21:131-144.
[39] Vinik AI, Silva MP, Woltering EA, et al. Biochemical testing for neuroendocrine tumors. *Pancreas.* 2009; 38:876-889. 93:1945-1948.
[40] Washington M, Tang L, Berlin J, et al. Protocol for the examination of specimens from patient with neuroendocrine tumors (carcinoid tumors) of the appendix. *Arch Pathol Lab Med.* 2010; 134:171-175.
[41] Washington M, Tang L, Berlin J, et al. Protocol for the examination of specimens from patient with neuroendocrine tumors (carcinoid tumors) of the colon and rectum. *Arch Pathol Lab Med.* 2010; 134:176-180.

[42] Washington M, Tang L, Berlin J, et al. Protocol for the examination of specimens from patient with neuroendocrine tumors (carcinoid tumors) of the small intestine and ampulla. *Arch Pathol Lab Med.* 2010; 134:181-186.
[43] Washington M, Tang L, Berlin J, et al. Protocol for the examination of specimens from patient with neuroendocrine tumors (carcinoid tumors) of the stomach. *Arch Pathol Lab Med.* 2010; 134:187-191.